Melanoma: Prevention, Detection, and Treatment

Melanoma

Prevention, Detection, and Treatment

Catherine M. Poole
with DuPont Guerry IV, M.D.

Drawings by David Low, M.D.

Yale University Press
New Haven & London

Published with assistance from the foundation established in memory of Philip Hamilton McMillan of the Class of 1894, Yale College.

The information and suggestions contained in this book are not intended to replace the services of your physician or caregiver. Because each person and medical situation is unique, you should consult your own physician to get answers to your personal questions, to evaluate any symptoms you may have, or to receive suggestions on appropriate medications.

The staging system for malignant melanoma of the skin reproduced here as Appendix A is used with the permission of the American Joint Committee on Cancer, Chicago, Illinois. The original source for this material is the AJCC *Manual for Staging of Cancer*, 4th edition (1992), published by J. B. Lippincott Company, Philadelphia.

The ads in Figure 26 are reprinted with permission from the American Academy of Dermatology. All rights reserved.

Photography by William K. Witmer, medical photographer, Pigmented Lesion Clinic.

Designed by James J. Johnson and set in Adobe Utopia with Syntax type by G & S Typesetters, Inc., Austin, Texas. Printed in the United States of America by Data Reproductions Corporation, Auburn Hills, Michigan.

Library of Congress Cataloging-in-Publication Data

Poole, Catherine M.
    Melanoma: Prevention, detection, and treatment / Catherine M. Poole, with DuPont Guerry IV.
        p.   cm.
    Includes index.
    ISBN 0-300-07361-5 (cloth : alk. paper).—ISBN 0-300-07362-3 (paper)

    1. Melanoma.   I. Guerry, DuPont, 1942– .   II. Title.
    RC280.M37P66   1998
    616.99'477—dc21   97-39658

A catalogue record for this book is available from the British Library.

The paper in this book meets the guidelines for permanence and durability of the Committee on Production Guidelines for Book Longevity of the Council on Library Resources.

10   9   8   7   6   5   4   3   2   1

To Wallace H. Clark, Jr., and the patients and staff of the University of Pennsylvania Pigmented Lesion Group, who have taught us how to look for and see curable melanomas.

D. G.

To those who are dealing with melanoma in their lives; and to the health care professionals who are dedicated to finding a way to prevent and treat melanoma successfully.

C. P.

Contents

Preface

Books about cancer seem always to begin with scary stories about people whose deaths could have been averted by its early detection and with statistics that describe the growing menace of the disease to the population. The accounts move on to grapple with the "causes" of lung or breast or colon or prostate cancer and eventually deal with related issues of prevention. The authors of such books may talk about genes as if they were fate (breast cancer is "caused" by one broken gene in some families) and about environmental factors as if they were inevitable executioners (a standard Western diet "causes" colon cancer).

Such books conclude with the promise that new research is about to deliver a novel and effective preventive strategy, a better diagnostic test, or a cure that does not involve surgery, radiation, and toxic chemicals. This new approach may rely on gene therapy or something "natural" and "biological."

These books do provide useful information—smoking really is bad for you and is a potent cause of lung cancer; mammography is a modestly effective tool in decreasing breast cancer mortality and should be widely and regularly used. But they usually promise too much, at least for the real world of the here and now; and they often get it wrong. They miss a number of cancer's features—its many forms, its multifactorial causality, its multiple mechanisms of growth and spread, and its complex interactions with the immune system and other systems that defend bodily integrity. The authors neglect to point out that targets on cancer cells for therapeutic attack are usually also present on normal cells and that agents to be used in prevention and therapy not only are intrinsically weak but also have side-effects.

Writers make these mistakes because they oversimplify, and often they oversimplify because they fail to recognize the subtlety and complexity of the causation and evolution of the disease. Cancer is best viewed as a diverse family of chronic diseases whose early manifestations gestate for years and are usually hidden from view—under the skin, in a duct of a breast, or in a segment of the bowel.

With help from me and colleagues, Catherine Poole has written a different book—or a book different in substance. She has adopted the sensible format of the generic cancer book. But because melanoma is unlike other malignancies in two specific ways, her discussion makes for a guide that has real utility now. Melanoma is different from other cancers because it is pigmented and because it arises in the top layer of the skin. Hence, it is distinctive and visible—apparent to our best-developed sense (sight) and "on" an organ of great psychosocial importance (see Chapter 2).

Melanoma is a book that delivers on the promise to teach information that will save lives. At its core, it is about how to detect melanoma when biologically it is still *early cancer*. By this I mean cancer at the first step in its evolution, when it is potentially detectable but still incapable of spreading to distant sites. It is such a colonization of tissues away from the tumor's point of origin, called metastasis, that is potentially death-dealing. Biologically early cancer is not to be underestimated, however. If left alone, it is liable to take the next step, at which metastasis becomes ever more likely with time.

Most cancers of all types begin with that first step, but in most it is invisible. In melanoma, however, it is easy to see as a distinctive, flat, brown or black pigmented spot on the skin, one that is often slowly but perceptibly changing (see Chapter 4) or that can be detected as change within a mole (see Chapter 3).

Melanomas discovered in this flat phase of their evolution are invariably cured, usually with simple, inexpensive, cosmetically uncomplicated outpatient surgery. And even the next step, the lumpy phase, is cured more often than not (70 percent of patients with melanoma that has reached this later step are cured with comparable surgery).

The trick, of course, is for you to learn to see early melanoma (the pictures in Chapter 2 are vivid and representative) and to figure out who needs particular and professional observation (again, see the core chapters, Chapters 3 and 4). Once you have mastered the routine of really looking at your skin (and that of people close to you), the chance of developing the potentially lethal step in melanoma will go from small to vanishingly small. Hence, you should be fearless about pointing out suspicious spots in others and about having your own evaluated and managed. Chapter 5 tells you how to do this.

Chapter 6 deals with disease that has escaped beyond the place of its origin (the primary site), a step in melanoma that will happen to some small but irreducible fraction of patients, no matter how good we all get at taking care of and watching our skin. This chapter conveys the important information that there is an initial step in metastasis when the disease has spread only to nearby lymph glands. At this step, cure still is a reasonable likelihood.

We also remind you that even serious disease can turn out well in some patients and that at least incremental advances are at hand in the "biological" therapy of disease that is at high risk of being metastatic. We can now see the glimmer of a promise of useful therapy for some patients with widespread disease.

Catherine closes with an important chapter on matters of the heart and soul (Chapter 7) and one on eradication of melanoma in what should be the best sense—the prevention of disease rather than its removal. Chapter 8 is about the avoidance of excessive sun exposure, particularly in childhood. It argues that with exposure to sunshine, moderation makes sense—it will promote healthier skin, will retard many of the changes in skin thought to reflect aging, and will greatly diminish the number of nonmelanoma skin cancers. It is also very likely to control the melanoma epidemic.

Catherine Poole is a practical, no-nonsense person. It is no surprise that she has written a practical, no-nonsense guide to how to deal with melanoma in the real world. She has had the disease herself, and this perspective lends her book authenticity and spirit.

DuPont Guerry IV, M.D.
Director, Melanoma Program
University of Pennsylvania
Comprehensive Cancer Center
Philadelphia, Pennsylvania

Acknowledgments

My children Jesse and Carey were the motivation for my writing this book. My primary mission is to educate people—and in so doing, help prevent melanoma from afflicting future generations. My friends provided continual reinforcement and reassurance as I worked on *Melanoma*.

I also hope to provide some comfort to those with melanoma. I know how frightening it is and how confusing the information you get about melanoma can be. I have spoken with many melanoma patients and read their letters, and I wish to thank them for their contribution to the book. I especially want to mention Nancy Cobourn, who told me the story of her father (Frank Styer), Sam Donaldson, who talked with me after his struggle with melanoma, and Lisa, who readily supplied me with the details of her battle with the disease. All were generous to share their stories, which appear in the first chapter.

I would also like to thank two of the most courageous women I know: Carolyn Marks and Lyn Carroll. They provide constant inspiration through their example in handling adversity.

Let me also take this opportunity to express my gratitude to all the extremely busy people who took the time to help me with this book: Richard Gallagher, a particularly caring epidemiologist, and David Low, who created the wonderful illustrations for the book. Also, I appreciate the assistance of Robin Holmes, who is a clinical specialist at the Pigmented Lesion Clinic, and Stephanie Waldman, Dr. Guerry's assistant.

Unless otherwise noted, all the quotations in the book are taken from personal interviews carried on between 1993 and 1997.

DuPont Guerry refers to this as "your book," but once in a while he slips and calls it "our" book. Despite his denial, this is *his* book too. He deserves much credit for his attention to medical accuracy, writing style, and selection of photographs and illustrations. He put numerous hours in on this project, even though he barely keeps his head above water with his commitments to research, teaching, and patients.

Going into this project, I thought I knew a lot about melanoma, but he has taught me humility in regard to my medical knowledge. Medicine, as I have learned, is an art, not a science. Dr. Guerry's opinions may therefore differ at times from those of other experts. This is the nature of intelligent interpretation of medical research—of which I had far too simplistic a view. His patients, colleagues, and I agree: not only is he a skilled clinician, but he has shown himself to be adept at healing the spirit too. He is a warm and generous human being.

Catherine Poole

1 Close Encounters with Melanoma

Cancer is feared more than death in our society. Melanoma seems especially ominous: "a malign, ingrown melanoma, spreading softly its dark tide."[1] In reality, melanoma *is* menacing because no sure or easy treatment for it exists once it has spread beyond the initial site. In this book we consider not only the diagnosis and treatment of the disease but also the steps you can take to protect yourself from getting melanoma in the first place—or to discover it before it becomes dangerous. To put the potential outcomes in perspective, it might be helpful to look at the impact of the disease on the lives of three people. The first story is my own (Catherine Poole's) and shows how I contended with a low-risk melanoma during pregnancy. The next is that of prominent news journalist Sam Donaldson, whose melanoma spread to a lymph node. Third is the story of Frank Styer, whose disease became so widespread that it took his life.

Catherine Poole   The holiday season was fading and so was I—I was five months pregnant and suffering from the flu. As a busy free-lance writer with an active toddler, I didn't often stretch out on the couch in my nightgown as I did that afternoon. For some reason, while lying on my side, I glanced at the back of my leg. To my surprise, a band of little black bubbles appeared to be growing out of what I had always thought was a birthmark. Instinctively I knew this was something to be concerned about. I had dealt with cancer a lot in my family, and its warning signs were familiar to me. This was definitely an "obvious change in a mole."

The next morning I went to a dermatologist. We were both pregnant, our bellies nearly brushing in the small examination room, and she had no room to hide her alarmed reaction to the suspicious growth on my leg. With gloved hands (which made me feel I was harboring something infectious), she carefully examined the rest of my skin. She called a surgeon to get me in for a biopsy right then and there.

After injecting a local anesthetic, the surgeon cut out the mole, along with some tissue underneath and around it, and closed the wound with a few stitches. The procedure was quick and painless.

Waiting for the answer from the hospital pathology department was torture. I felt that my existence hinged on the results. As the days wore on, I couldn't eat or sleep. I was anxious about losing my pregnancy or, worse, dying and abandoning my newborn and two-year-old.

After two weeks of suspense, I finally called and urged the surgeon to send the biopsy to a teaching hospital in Philadelphia for a faster answer. In less than twenty-four hours, Wallace Clark, a pathologist at the University of Pennsylvania, determined that it was melanoma.

When the dermatologist called me with the news, I felt disembodied as she sympathetically advised surgery and suggested that I see a specialist in Philadelphia. I then called my family doctor, also a friend, for a list of surgeons. His voice faltered, making him sound more upset than I was about the diagnosis (this was totally out of character for him). The reactions of both doctors really sent me into a panic. Next I called my nurse-midwife. She sounded worried, too. But she provided reassurance when she read to me from one of her nursing texts about melanoma. The book said that women often have a better prognosis than men, especially with a melanoma located on a lower extremity. That tiny piece of information kept my spirits up for a long time.

I needed more information, though, and I obtained it from the National Cancer Institute Cancer Information Service Hotline (800-4-CANCER), which had also helped my sister learn more about her breast cancer. The hotline supplied a list of melanoma specialists in the Philadelphia area. (Note: the hotline no longer provides physician referrals; instead, it offers a list of research and teaching facilities.) I had a choice of two doctors: the first was DuPont Guerry; the other was the one my dermatologist had mentioned.

I still wasn't sure about my prognosis and didn't know exactly what treatment I needed. Hoping to find out, I made an appointment with the physician at the teaching hospital recommended by my dermatologist. As my husband waited with me to see the doctor, I noticed him looking very

worried for the first time. At last he was validating my feelings of anxiety.

My husband was allowed into the examination room
with me. I wanted him there to help remember the details.
Although I felt on top of things with my list of prepared
questions, my mind seemed shrouded in a fog at times.
Sometimes I would ask a question and not even listen to
the answer.

I liked the doctor—he was kind, and willing to discuss
everything in great detail. I was relieved when he suggested
further surgery that could be performed at our local hospital: a simple procedure of taking additional skin around the
site of the melanoma to ensure that all the malignant cells
had been removed. From the pathology report, he surmised
that I had an 80 percent chance of surviving eight years,
whereas Wallace Clark's estimate on my pathology report
had been 95 percent. I liked Clark's odds better, but I wanted
100 percent!

The next hurdle was to find a surgeon quickly, since the
doctors were acting as if there was some urgency. The surgeon I chose was bright, young, and flexible about my terms:
local anesthesia, no extended hospital stay, and no drugs
that might compromise my pregnancy. This doctor was very
cheerful about my prognosis—saying, "These things rarely
ever come back." (I had him repeat this to me every so often.) He and I worked together as a team during the whole
process.

I agreed to a wide excision. The surgeon took a two-
centimeter (three-quarter-inch) strip of skin around the
biopsy scar—more than needed to be removed. (Had I read
this book first, it would have been half that.) I had to have a

skin graft from my hip to close the wound. The worst part of being awake for the surgery was the sound of the planer that was used. It sounded like a chain saw as it vibrated through my whole body, shimming off a piece of skin to be grafted onto my leg.

My recuperation was steady, and the deadline I had to meet for a magazine cover story kept me sane. The pain from the skin graft was the worst part. I also found it difficult, in my pregnant state, to adjust to walking on crutches. A particular challenge was to get to the bathroom gracefully in the middle of the night. One night, after gathering up my crutches in the dark, I tripped over my husband's shoes and fell flat on my face.

A few months later I returned to the teaching hospital for a follow-up examination. This visit was upsetting because I wasn't able to see the same doctor, even after requesting him in advance, and no family members were permitted in the examination room. The final blow came when this doctor told me that I should not plan to breastfeed my baby. The following day I called the Pigmented Lesion Clinic at the University of Pennsylvania and spoke with one of the nurses, Jean Thompson.

She assured me that breastfeeding would not make my disease reappear, as the other doctor had insinuated. Jean's reassurance, coupled with Dr. Clark's pathology report, influenced me to switch to the clinic.

At almost nine months pregnant, I didn't feel like going anywhere too far from home. I had gained forty pounds and couldn't even bend over to plug in a fan. But we made the trip to Philadelphia to meet DuPont Guerry, one of the doctors recommended by the Cancer Hotline.

The Pigmented Lesion Clinic was housed in a drab old building with stained linoleum hallways. The elevator was not to be trusted. We could hardly concentrate on a conversation because the television in the waiting room was blaring a soap opera. Despite the tacky appearance of the place, we found a warm, family-oriented staff who welcomed my husband and daughter into the examination room.

DuPont Guerry talked so fast that he nearly erased his slight southern drawl. And despite his rush to get to his next patient, he was willing to answer all my questions. His prognosis was confusing and filled with statistics, but I did understand his reassurance that I was likelier to get killed on the Schuylkill Expressway than by my melanoma.

In taking my history, Dr. Guerry asked if I had had many sunburns as a child. I recalled growing up in Arizona and having my mother on several occasions soothe my sun-scorched skin by dabbing it with cotton soaked in iced tea. I also remembered dreading our family vacations at the beach. I always had to stay fully clothed, because otherwise I would burn badly even when I was up to my neck in the ocean.

Dr. Guerry explained that if the unlikely happened and the melanoma in my system spread, I would probably find it in the lymph nodes in my groin area, most likely within the next two to three years. I was to return in three months to get a chest X-ray after my baby was born.

A few weeks later, a ten-pound boy was born, apparently unscathed by my tangle with melanoma. I couldn't forget about the incident just yet, though. My surgeon had issued a directive to my midwife to have the placenta sectioned by

Pathology at the local hospital. As he explained in his letter, the pathology needed to be performed because melanoma is one of the few cancers that can cross the placenta and affect the fetus. After Dr. Guerry assured me that this result had been reported only in cases where the mother had widespread melanoma, I declined to have this step performed.

I returned to Dr. Guerry a few months later for an extensive work-up. It was slightly humiliating to have the clinic's photographer take pictures of my naked postpartum body from head to toe, with a close-up of my "funny-looking" mole. Dr. Guerry explained that the photos would enable the physicians on subsequent visits to look for changes that might herald a second melanoma.

At one of my recent visits, Dr. Guerry said, after examining me, "Now get out of here, because you're too damned healthy to be here." That meant a lot to me; I knew the potentially dire consequences of a recurrence. I've been fortunate enough to remain healthy and free of melanoma for the past eight years.

Sam Donaldson According to Sam Donaldson, he "had always, or for many, many years, had a mole on the inside of my ankle near the bone." (All quotations of Sam Donaldson in this chapter are taken from my notes of a personal interview with him on December 16, 1996.) It wasn't until a vacation with his wife in 1988 that they both noticed a peculiar look to the mole. It had changed colors—it was blue around the edges and brown in the center and looked very inflamed. When they returned to Washington, Sam headed straight to his family doctor to get the mole checked. The doctor was concerned too, so Sam entered the hospital to have the mole excised. The surgeon took a wide band of skin around the mole and quite a bit of underlying tissue close to the bone. Sam had several stitches and had to stay off the foot for three weeks or more.

According to the first pathology report, the sample was benign. But his doctor was still suspicious and shipped it off to two more pathologists, including one in Boston. They too reported that the mole was benign. Sam, relieved, soon forgot about the whole ordeal.

Seven and a half years later while Sam was showering, he found a lump the size of an egg in his groin. This time he went to an internist, who thought the swollen node might indicate some sort of infection. When Sam told him about the removal of the mole, the doctor sent him to a surgical oncologist that very day. The surgeon speculated that it was melanoma that had spread from the mole removed from his ankle.

Next, Sam was directed to have a biopsy of the enlarged lymph node and a CAT scan to determine whether the melanoma had spread anywhere else in his body. In the meantime, the surgeon arranged for Sam to be seen by Steven Rosenberg, chief of surgery at the National Cancer Institute (NCI) and a highly regarded melanoma researcher.

When NCI's pathologists reviewed the slides of Sam's original lesion, they had no question that it was melanoma. After viewing the results of the CAT scan and examining Sam, Dr. Rosenberg told him that he had a good chance of living a long, normal life. Sam didn't believe him; he had convinced himself otherwise. Sam says, "I realize that all cancers aren't a death sentence, but you know some are worse than others, and melanoma is the Tyrannosaurus rex of cancers." He figured that he only had a few months to live. But Rosenberg persisted in his optimism. He said that there was no evidence of involvement in other areas of the body. Given that it also had been a long time since the original lesion had appeared, it seemed probable that his body was effectively confining the melanoma.

Sam proceeded to have the adjacent lymph nodes surgically removed by Dr. Rosenberg. The pathology report confirmed that no additional lymph nodes were involved. This meant that Sam had a Stage III melanoma, and about a 50 percent chance of being cured. As soon as he recuperated, Sam started looking for additional melanoma therapies that might raise his odds. He called Dr. John Kirkwood in Pittsburgh to check out taking alpha-interferon—but then decided against it. Sam says, "I'm sixty-two, and when I drag myself to bed at night in some hotel after shooting *Prime Time* all day, I think I should be thirty-two. I can't afford the loss of energy that this treatment causes. Only if I lost energy for a year and it would buy me the rest of my life would I go for it."

Sam insists that he "will never look back on that decision. If this melanoma returns, I'm not going to say that I should have had this or that treatment."

Sam was still free of disease, after two years, in June 1997. In the meantime, he remarks, "I certainly have developed a better personal understanding of people who have cancer or an illness, and I'm adopting a slower pace of life. I'm not sure if it's due to the aging process or to the melanoma. Maybe it is a little of both."

Frank Styer At age sixty-three, Frank had finally reached a well-deserved retirement. He had worked hard since his youth, first on the family farm and then overseeing maintenance for a private school in the small rural township where he lived. His outdoor occupation brought him a high dose of sunshine over the years, and with his blonde hair, blue eyes, and fair skin, he had a strong tendency to burn.

As his daughter Nancy told me, "He had never been sick a day in his life until he needed an appendectomy that year of his retirement." A couple months after that, he complained to his family doctor about a lump on his neck. The doctor thought it was a sebaceous cyst and sent him to a surgeon, who concurred.

Frank was told not to worry about it but to come back in six months if it didn't go away. The cyst regressed a bit and then became inflamed, so Frank returned to the surgeon. When the lump was removed, the pathology report told a much different story: it was melanoma. Frank explained to the doctor that there had been a mole where the lump developed but that his barber had nicked it and then shaved it off a few years earlier. Nevertheless, the doctors made an extensive and fruitless search for the primary source of the melanoma. Frank and his family met with the head of a melanoma program at a medical school to see whether he might participate in a clinical trial, but the doctor said that no such study was available for him at that time.

A few months later, CAT scans located a tumor in his chest. Once the tumor had been removed, the pathology report described it as a lymph node filled with melanoma. Over the next two years, Frank suffered immensely, riding a physical and emotional roller coaster. He endured frequent scans and surgery, as well as the side-effects of chemotherapy.

The surgeon chased the melanoma from the bladder to the adrenal glands, but it kept reappearing. Frank died at home three years after beginning his struggle with melanoma.

Melanoma can run the gamut from innocuous to deadly, depending in large part on whether it is caught early on. Once it has spread to distant parts of the body, it seems to defy the toxic chemicals and aggressive treatments that keep some other cancers in check.

By reading further, you can learn *now* how to spot an early melanoma and therefore lessen your risk of developing a more dangerous form of the disease, and you can discover how to decrease the chances of your children's ever having to deal with melanoma.

2 What Is Melanoma?

Each hour one person in the United States dies from melanoma—Press release from AAD 1996 Melanoma/ Skin Cancer Detection and Prevention Campaign.

Melanoma was known at the time of Hippocrates, who referred to it as a black tumor. It was first reported in Western medical literature by John Hunter, an English physician, in 1787. Hunter documented and preserved a melanoma tumor taken from a thirty-five-year-old man's lower jaw. The melanoma reappeared three years later, a recurrence thought to have been triggered during a drunken brawl when the man's chin was struck with a stick. (Doctors now believe that hitting or rubbing a melanoma has little effect on how it behaves.) Dr. Hunter described the lump as "soft and black" and labeled it a "cancerous fungous excrescence." In 1968, a U.S. pathologist confirmed that the specimen preserved at a medical museum in England was a melanoma.[1]

Since Hunter's time, we have had no shortage of melanoma cases. In fact, the ever-increasing incidence of melanoma among whites worldwide began with forced emigration of sun-sensitive Englishmen to an Australian penal colony in the late 1870s. Many other English citizens, lured by prospects of new fortune, followed on their heels. Thanks to the conjunction of its fair-skinned immigrant population and the equatorial sun, Australia has the dubious distinction of having the highest melanoma rate in the world today.

In the early 1900s, the United States experienced a sweeping tide of radical social change. Society loosened up, and fashion followed the shift in attitude: more skin was bared. No longer could women stand being shackled by ankle-length dresses that dragged in the dirt or got tangled in a car's stick shift and pedals. Meanwhile, men took to wearing shorter collars and sleeves, and some shaved their beards and mustaches and eventually found it acceptable to go shirtless in the summer sun. Within a few decades, pallor was no longer fashionable; suntans had come into vogue. The historical trend toward increased sun exposure may help explain the upswing in melanoma rates.[2]

Your Body's Largest Organ   To understand what melanoma is and how it develops, it is helpful to understand basic anatomy and the function of the skin. Generally, skin isn't considered a functioning organ like the liver or the brain. Actually, most people don't realize that their skin is an organ at all. They understand that it protects them from external stimuli—but not that they need to protect *it*.

The skin is, however, the largest organ of the body, responsible for shielding the rest of the body from excessive light and extreme temperatures. The skin also has the important job of guarding the body from infection and injury.

The skin's secondary role is social. Pathologist Wallace Clark refers to the skin as the "cosmetic organ of our bodies." Because it is one of the major ways humans present themselves to others, they work hard to adorn or improve their skin, by applying makeup to it, having it pierced, or undergoing plastic surgery.

Yet human skin can't compare with the hides of the rest of the animal kingdom; according to Dr. Clark, "Even were you to be arrayed with less spectacular creatures such as the . . . spotted skunk, the unadorned skin of *Homo sapiens* is, by comparison, a scenic disaster."[3]

Any animal's epidermis not only serves an esthetic function but provides an extra layer of protection from the sun. According to Dr. Clark, our skin structure is closest to pigs', for "only swine have the same organization of the dermis (inner layer of skin) as humans. Also like humans, swine enjoy lying in the sun, tan in response to the sun, and will drink beer in large quantities."[4]

Human skin is made up of two layers: the epidermis, or outer layer; and the dermis, or inner layer. Below the dermis is the fatty, or subcutaneous, layer (subcutis). The dermis is divided into an upper part, called the papillary dermis, and a lower part called the reticular dermis. The dermis contains several different types of cells and fibrous tissues, along with blood and lymph vessels that nourish the epidermis. This outer layer, the epidermis, is where most skin cancers evolve. (See Figure 1.)

In the lower region of the epidermis are the melanocytes, cells that make a dark pigment called melanin, which contributes to skin coloring. Melanocytes feed the melanin pigment to cells above them, called keratinocytes. This provides

Figure 1. Skin Structure: A Cross-Section of Human Skin

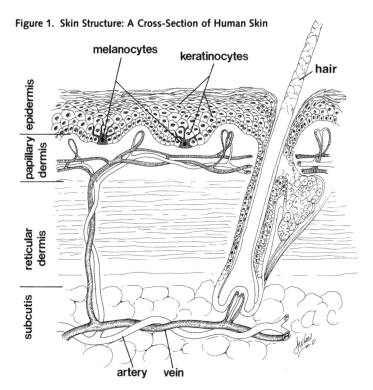

Melanocytes sit at the bottom of the epidermis and feed melanin pigment to a group of client keratinocytes.

them and the underlying structures with a natural sunblock of sorts. Melanoma is the uncontrolled growth of melanocytes in one spot, thought to be set off by some of the ultraviolet wavelengths in sunlight (and sometimes other influences).

If left to its natural course, a melanoma can eventually penetrate from the epidermis into the dermis and adapt to growing there. Once melanoma spreads to the dermis, it has access to blood and lymph vessels—the freeways to the rest of the body. Therefore, if the melanoma reaches the dermis and is able to flourish, its cells have the potential to spread to other areas of the body. The dermis is the setting where melanoma takes on its role as a full-fledged malignancy.

What Is Melanoma?   Melanoma is a form of skin cancer not to be confused with the more common squamous cell or basal cell skin cancers. These very common skin cancers arise from keratinocytes in the epidermis and are also triggered by sun exposure—yet seldom become life threatening. In contrast, melanoma, according to Dr. Guerry, is made up of the "malign progeny of melanocytes" and has a much higher potential to spread to other parts of your body and become a life-threatening illness.

There are several different types of melanoma. Superficial spreading melanoma is the most common type of melanoma, making up 70 to 80 percent of all cases. (See Plate 1.) Although it is found most frequently on women's legs and on the backs of people of both sexes, it can arise anywhere on the body, including areas never exposed to the sun. Superficial spreading melanoma often develops from an existing mole, but it can also come from an unblemished bit of skin. It looks like a brown-black spreading stain, usually at least half a centimeter (about a quarter of an inch) in diameter.

Nodular melanoma accounts for 10 percent of melanoma cases. (See Plate 2, Figure 6.) It is found in the same locations as superficial spreading melanoma, is a bit more common in men than in women, and also frequently arises from a mole.

It is raised and dome-shaped and sometimes resembles a blood-blister. Both nodular and superficial spreading melanomas appear to be triggered by the combination of excessive intermittent sun exposure and skin sensitivity, as evidenced, for example, in sunburns.

Lentigo maligna melanoma (see Plate 2, Figure 7) is less common than either of the other two and is usually seen in older people. It is most commonly found on the face and other parts of the body that are chronically exposed to the sun. It develops after many years of heavy sun exposure and first appears as a dark and irregularly shaped stain. Lentigo maligna melanoma does not develop from moles.

Most of the melanomas already mentioned appear predominantly in white people, whereas acral lentiginous melanoma occurs in approximately the same low frequency among whites and in people of color. (See Plate 2, Figure 8.) It appears most frequently on the palms of the hands or the soles of the feet, on the undersurface of the fingers or toes, and under the nails. When it affects the nail, the melanoma begins at the base and makes a streak that extends to the tip of the nail. The thumbs and great toes are most often affected.

Acral lentiginous melanoma is not attributed to sun exposure. This is the type of melanoma that killed reggae music star Bob Marley in 1981. According to the *Philadelphia Inquirer,* he had acral lentiginous melanoma of his big toe, which spread to his lungs and brain.[5]

Mucosal melanoma appears on the mucous membranes of the body—inside the mouth and in the anal-genital region. It is a rare form of melanoma whose cause is unknown but which, given its location, is also unrelated to sun exposure.

Another uncommon melanoma arises at the back of the eye. Its cause, too, is unclear, since this area is protected by the cornea and lens from the harmful wavelengths of sunlight. Even so, medical investigators speculate that ultraviolet radiation, especially in childhood, may pass through the front of the eye and trigger this rare kind of melanoma later in life.

Exceptionally, melanomas of all kinds can present themselves as amelanotic (without melanin pigment). These melanomas are difficult to recognize because they don't have the characteristic darkness of melanoma but rather show up as pink or red growths.

Plates 1 through 4 (containing Figures 2 through 20) show what melanoma looks like.

When Melanoma Becomes Malignant

A melanoma isn't born malignant; in other words, it doesn't possess the ability to spread to the internal organs until it has progressed through certain growth phases. Dr. Wallace Clark coined the term *radial growth phase.* (See Figure 21 and Chapter 4.) In this phase, the melanoma is nontumorigenic—that is, it doesn't form a tumor or lump or nodule. This phase actually comprises two steps: in the first the melanoma cells are contained entirely in the epidermis. The cancer is thus described by the Latin term *in situ,* meaning "in place." In the second step, the invasive radial growth phase, the melanoma cells may barely invade the dermis but do not flourish there. At this step the cancer is no longer regarded as being in situ. During the radial growth phase, the melanoma can't send out cells to

Plate 1
Superficial Spreading Melanomas

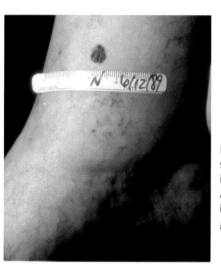

Figure 2. An early melanoma of the superficial spreading type on the inside of a woman's lower right leg. Although invasive, this melanoma is still at an early step (the radial growth phase).

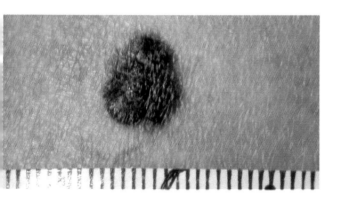

Figure 3. A close-up of the early melanoma shown in Figure 2 (the ruler shows millimeters). This and the lesion shown in Figure 5 have the ABCDE's of early melanoma—asymmetry, border irregularity, color variation (here black, pinkish gray, and shades of brown), a diameter greater than six millimeters (about the diameter of a pencil eraser), and sometimes elevation. Melanoma also often perceptibly increases in diameter.

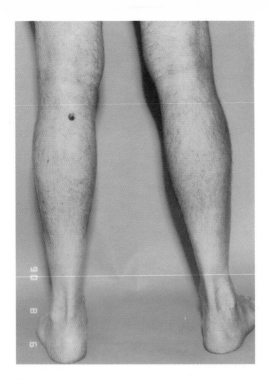

Figure 4. A superficial spreading melanoma on the back of a man's leg. Although women are especially likely to develop melanomas in this spot, men can too. Remember to look at the back of your body when you do your skin examination.

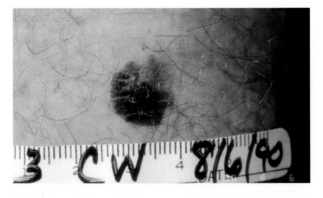

Figure 5. A close-up of the lesion shown in Figure 4. This melanoma shows a small vertical growth phase, which although not apparent to the eye, has some chance of metastasizing.

Plate 2
Other Forms of Melanomas of the Skin

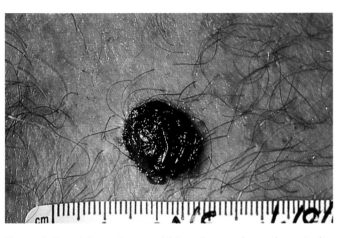

Figure 6. A nodular melanoma. This melanoma has only vertical growth phase without any apparent earlier radial growth phase. It started as a small coal-black lump that grew in just a few months to the size shown.

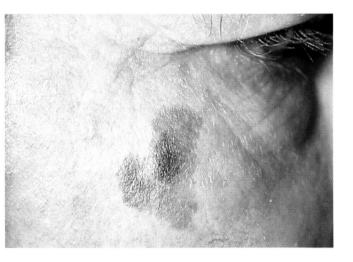

Figure 7. A lentigo maligna melanoma on the right cheek of an older man. This is an early melanoma of the kind that is associated with a lifetime of intense sun exposure and sun damage. It is a pure radial growth phase melanoma.

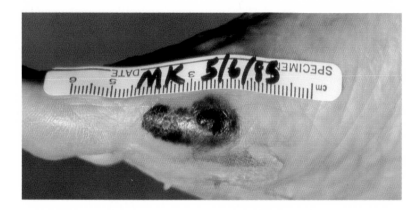

Figure 8. An acral lentiginous melanoma on the inside of the right foot. This is a rare form of melanoma that is not associated with sun exposure and occurs with the same low frequency in all races. The lesion shown here has both radial and vertical growth phases. The shiny black lump within the flat portion of the right side of the lesion is the vertical growth phase.

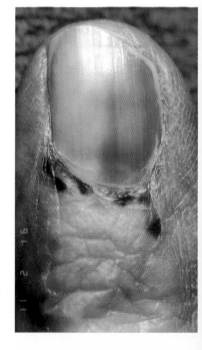

Figure 9. A subungual melanoma. This is a form of acral lentiginous melanoma that grows under the base of a nail and discolors it, usually in a broad, irregular band of pigment that extends from the base of the nail to its tip. Unlike nail discoloration due to trauma (caused, for example, by hammer blows to a thumb or by pressure from poorly fitting running shoes on great toes), the pigment does not slowly grow out to leave an ever widening clear zone above the base of the nail. Here, dark pigment is also seen in the skin around the base of the nail.

Plate 3
Ordinary and Congenital Moles

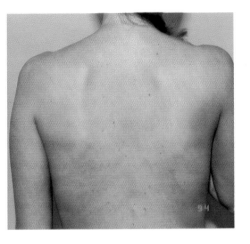

Figure 10. The upper back of a thirty-five-year-old with scattered ordinary moles. (Look particularly between the shoulder blades.)

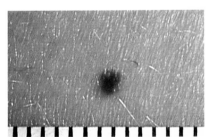

Figure 11. A tiny ordinary flat mole.

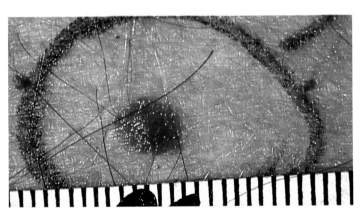

Figure 12. A small ordinary domed mole.

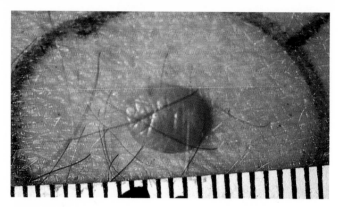

Figure 13. A large ordinary domed mole that lost most of its pigment.

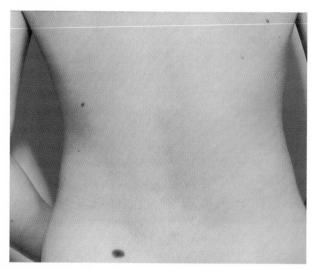

Figure 14. The back of a fourteen-year-old with a few ordinary moles and a small congenital mole over the pelvic bone to the left of the midline.

Figure 15. A close-up of the congenital mole shown in Figure 14. This lesion grew as the patient grew. It is slightly raised and has a pebbly texture with some speckles of darker pigment. The patient and her parents have decided not to remove this mole but to check it by sight and by feel monthly.

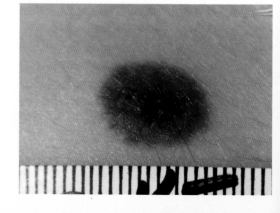

Plate 4
Dysplastic Moles

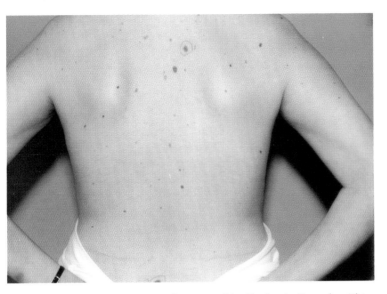

Figure 16. The back of a twenty-five-year-old with dysplastic moles. This patient has both more than the average number of ordinary moles and a few moles that are unusual (for example, the mole to the left of the shoulder blade that is circled and designated 1).

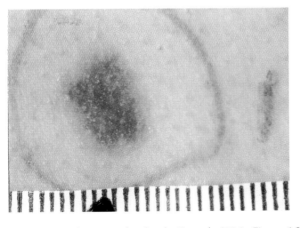

Figure 17. A close-up of a dysplastic mole (#1 in Figure 16). This mole is dysplastic because it has fuzzy, indistinct, irregular borders, is several shades of brown, and is flat throughout and large (its long diameter is more than five millimeters).

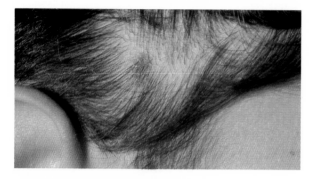

Figure 18. A dysplastic mole on the scalp that is flat throughout. Dysplastic scalp moles have the same tiny chance of giving rise to melanomas as dysplastic moles elsewhere, but they may be more difficult to keep an eye on because they are hidden by hair. If they are too difficult to follow for change, they should be removed.

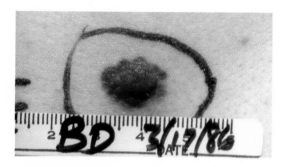

Figure 19. A dysplastic mole of the "fried egg" type. This mole looks like a sunny-side-up fried egg, with a normal, domed part in the center and a flat part. The flat part is where characteristic abnormalities are seen under the microscope.

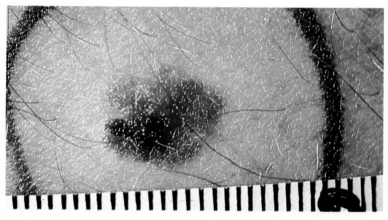

Figure 20. A dysplastic mole in which a melanoma appeared, one of many dysplastic moles in a patient with a past history of melanoma. When he reported that this mole had developed an area of darkness, it was photographed and removed.

Figure 21. Radial and Vertical Growth Phases of Melanoma

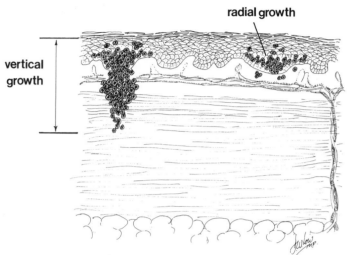

The two phases in the growth of primary melanomas: in the radial growth phase, melanoma cells may enter the top part of the dermis, but they do not grow to produce a lump (tumor) there. In the vertical growth phase the melanoma (here emerging from the radial growth phase in the epidermis) forms a tumor in the dermis and may extend into the subcutaneous tissue. The double arrow shows how tumor thickness is measured.

other parts of the body; still, if not recognized and removed, it will commonly proceed to the next step.

The next step is called the vertical growth, or tumorigenic, phase. The melanoma begins to grow as a tumor in the dermis, an expanding sphere made up of abnormal melanocytes. At this step, there is some chance that the cancer may spread. To prevent it from becoming fatal, it is essential to obliterate the growth while it is in its flat (radial growth) phase, before the lumpy (vertical growth) phase.

According to Dr. Guerry, "about a third of our patients who come to us with invasive melanomas have pure radial growth phase melanoma and can expect a cure rate indistinguishable from 100%. In our database [at the Pigmented Lesion Clinic], fully 87% of melanomas had at least a component of radial growth phase. This phase precedes the vertical phase and ought to be found and treated before the next step happens. The trick is to detect the features of early melanoma and act on them." [6]

To catch melanoma while it is still in its early phases, it is important to know the "look" of the lesion and understand the importance of any changes in it. The changes to look for are spelled out in the ABCD's of melanoma: asymmetry, border irregularity, color variation, and a diameter greater than six millimeters. Because with some early melanomas the skin is also slightly elevated or thickened, we can add an E for "elevation" to the ABCD's. (For more on the ABCDE's of melanoma, see Chapter 4.) If you know the topography of your skin and your loved ones' skin, you will be able to recognize melanoma before it progresses too far.

3 Who Gets Melanoma and Why

More than a century ago, William Norris, an English doctor, described certain similarities that he found among the melanoma patients he treated. He noted that most of his patients had light-colored hair and fair complexions, that their melanomas seemed to grow out of moles, and that patients' family members sometimes also had melanoma. Today, doctors look at the same factors to gauge who stands an increased risk of getting melanoma.[1]

Epidemiologists have pinpointed certain characteristics that, whether they occur separately or in conjunction, predict who is likely to get melanoma. These include:

- a sun-sensitive skin type that may freckle easily
- a history of spending too much time in the sun
- lots of common moles or any "funny-looking" (dysplastic) moles
- a personal or family history of any of the common kinds of skin cancer (squamous and basal cell carcinoma)
- a personal or family history of melanoma[2]

Other less important yet influential factors that seem to affect the development of melanoma are the person's gender, geographical location, and age. In a recent lecture, Dr. Allan Halpern, chief of dermatology at Memorial Sloan-Kettering Cancer Center, stated: "The risk associated with each factor is in itself not great; however, individuals who possess multiple melanoma risk factors may be at dramatically increased risk."

The Role of the Sun and Ultraviolet Radiation

The sun emits three types of electromagnetic radiation of concern to us: visible, ultraviolet (UV), and infrared. Visible radiation is the light we see; infrared is the radiation we feel warmth from; the invisible UV radiation seems to have the greatest potential for deleterious biological effects.

Ultraviolet radiation is divided into three wave bands: UV-A, UV-B, and UV-C. Only UV-A and UV-B reach the earth's surface and can therefore directly assault your skin. Ultraviolet radiation is a carcinogen, capable of both initiating a malignancy and promoting its growth and evolution. Although UV-B is thought to be the major carcinogenic agent in the formation of melanoma as well as nonmelanoma cancers, UV-A also makes a contribution. Light in both wave bands produces sunburn, along with the resultant skin damage, and accelerates the skin changes associated with aging, such as wrinkling and loss of elasticity.

Melanin pigment in the skin serves a protective role by absorbing and detoxifying ultraviolet radiation. The sensitivity of different skin types to sunburn and other photo-damaging effects is significantly related to how melanin is packaged and distributed in skin cells—factors that also largely determine skin type and color.

Which Skin Types Are Susceptible to Melanoma?

Melanoma affects almost exclusively people with white skin; the only important exception, as mentioned in Chapter 2, is acral lentiginous melanoma, which affects people of all skin colors and bears no relation to sun exposure. Freckles are an important barometer of both sun sensitivity and sun damage. A person who freckles easily has about twice the risk of getting melanoma of someone with no scattering of the telltale dots.

Some people have skin so sensitive that it turns a flaming shade of red when exposed to the sun for even a brief time. Usually their hair is red or blonde and their skin porcelain white. (It is possible, though, to have dark hair and very fair skin.)

Such skin, known as Type 1, is the most likely to develop melanoma. There are four skin types, determined by tanning ability. The following classification describes the untanned skin's reaction after being exposed to the sun, unprotected, for forty-five minutes to an hour. You probably know whether you tan well or not—and consequently can determine your skin type.

- Type 1 skin always burns, freckles readily, and is the most likely to develop melanoma.
- Type 2 usually burns and freckles, and it tans lighter than average. It also is susceptible to melanoma.

- Type 3 sometimes burns, tans about average, and is less vulnerable to melanoma than the first two types.
- Type 4 tans very readily and never burns; it develops melanoma less frequently than the three other types.

What Type of Sun Exposure Causes Melanoma?

The most common kinds of melanoma (superficial spreading and nodular) have been shown to be associated with heavy intermittent exposure to the sun, of the type that occurs, for example, when a person spends most of the time indoors but gets heavy doses of sun on vacations and weekends. Ultraviolet radiation from sunlight not only burns the skin but also affects the DNA, the genetic material, in the skin cells. Ultraviolet radiation may also have other far-reaching consequences, such as suppression of some function of the immune system.

Although intermittent, intense exposure of untanned skin to sunlight is an important risk factor for superficial spreading melanoma and nodular melanoma, it is not the only kind of sun exposure that poses a threat. Lentigo maligna melanoma is associated with long-term exposure to the sun. This kind of melanoma often afflicts older people—especially men—who have heavily sun-damaged skin. It commonly occurs on the face and ears.

Most dermatologists advise against relying on "artificial sunlight" to get a tan. The light tubes in tanning salons produce UV-A, a wavelength of light that is implicated in making skin look old and in causing nonmelanoma skin cancers. This kind of light may also collude with UV-B to trigger melanoma. Also, a UV-A tan does not protect against UV-B damage. That is, a "base tan" obtained at a tanning booth won't protect you from burning when you go outdoors.

Many dermatologists maintain that "bottled," or chemically colored, tans are the only safe tans. Commercial tanning formulas work by dying the top layers of the skin and affect only the dead cells. Nevertheless, bottled tans are no substitute for sun protection.

Is All Sun Exposure Bad?   Mild exposure to the sun is not harmful for most people. Indeed, it may have beneficial effects: it helps to activate vitamin D. It can also lift the spirits. It has been reported that the sort of mild, continual sun exposure that produces a bit of a tan but no burn may even protect you from melanoma. This modest protection comes at some cost, however. Tanning ages the skin and can precipitate nonmelanoma skin cancers.

Melanoma appears rarely in childhood, but heavy intermittent sun exposure early in life may cause melanoma to appear later, in adulthood. Like smoking, heavy exposure to sunlight causes delayed damage. Even if you start smoking when you are young, you won't generally get lung cancer before middle age.[3]

Melanoma occurs frequently among young adults; 35 percent of all cases are diagnosed in people younger than forty-five. Occurrences of melanoma peak among people in their fifties. The greatest overall rate of increase is seen in men, particularly men over sixty-five, according to the American Cancer Society's 1994 pamphlet, "Facts on Skin Cancer."

What Are Moles?   In the medical world moles are referred to as nevi (singular *nevus*). A
white adult may count an average of about twenty-five moles,
with the heaviest concentration in areas of the body where
the skin has had heavy intermittent exposure to sunlight.
Moles are a risk factor for melanoma regardless of skin type.
The predisposition to develop a great many moles may be
partly hereditary. Most children are born without moles, but
some acquire them as they grow older, from about age three
on. In a study published in July 1995, Richard Gallagher and
his colleagues at the British Columbia Cancer Agency found
a direct correlation between a history of childhood sunburns
and a high number of acquired nevi in children.[4]

Apparently, the skin forms moles as a reaction to sun
exposure. It may even be that moles protect sun-damaged
melanocytes within them, thus acting as little dark para-
sols to shade those patches of skin from further assault by
the sun.

A mole will usually first appear in childhood, as a small,
flat, tan to dark brown dot the size of a pinhead. It may then
slowly enlarge to become a round or oval growth, which may
be either flat or domed, usually smaller in diameter than a
standard pencil eraser. Moles may grow paler as a person
matures, and the raised ones often flatten out and eventually disappear late in life.

Some moles have nothing to do with sun exposure. At
birth about 1 percent of children have a single mole. These
congenital nevi are tan to dark brown, flat or slightly raised,
and may be greater than a centimeter (nearly half an inch) in
diameter. Such moles tend to expand as a person grows and
will often sprout hairs.

Although some doctors recommend eventual removal of these relatively common congenital nevi to prevent melanoma, the number that develop into melanoma is very small. Of course, parents or children may decide to have the moles removed for cosmetic reasons. Surgical removal is a simple routine procedure. Another option is lifelong monthly inspections of congenital moles, which should be closely watched for changes in color and palpated for changes in texture (thickening, for example). It is safe to shave hair associated with some of these moles, and cover-up cosmetics do no harm.

Giant congenital nevi, or garment nevi, which cover a significant portion of the body, are fortunately a rare occurrence in children. These moles carry a melanoma risk of 5 to 10 percent, and removal, even by expert plastic surgeons, is very difficult because of the moles' size and depth. Patients with garment nevi require expert consultation and a lifetime of follow-up care, including psychological support. (See the listing in Appendix B of a support group for people with garment nevi.)

Although most people have moles that are round and small, about 15 percent of the white population have funny-looking moles, referred to by practitioners as dysplastic nevi. They are also called atypical moles. (There is some disagreement as to the proper terminology. In 1992, the National Institute of Health Consensus Development Conference recommended calling them atypical moles, but *dysplastic moles* is a more precise term, which refers to the specific set of abnormalities that characterizes these moles.)

Dysplastic nevi are different from common moles because they are larger, at least five millimeters across, and either are flat throughout or look like a sunny-side-up fried egg (flat with a central dome). They are often variegated, in shades of brown and even pink, and usually have fuzzy, irregular borders. (See Chapter 2 for photos of dysplastic nevi.) They can be found even on parts of the body that haven't received much sun exposure, such as the buttocks of people of both sexes and the breasts of women, as well as on more exposed parts of the body.

It is important to pay attention to moles, because people with any dysplastic nevi or many ordinary moles have a higher risk of getting melanoma than those without them. Melanomas are frequently "born" in a mole, but you have to balance this information with the fact that any one mole, whether ordinary or dysplastic, is *very* unlikely to develop into melanoma.

We have to think about moles in two ways: first, as risk markers, and second, as potential precursors of melanoma. With regard to risk, the presence of many moles or of a few dysplastic moles tells you that you are perhaps two to seven times more likely to get melanoma sometime in your life than the average person with few ordinary moles and no dysplastic moles. In this case, moles tell you that your skin bears watching and warrants protecting. From another perspective, moles and dysplastic moles can be harbingers of melanoma. In 25 to 30 percent of cases, remnants of a preexisting mole are seen by the pathologist examining a melanoma under the microscope. But because there are so many moles out there and relatively few melanomas, the chance that any one mole will become a melanoma is comfortably small. Even in families with a high genetic tendency toward melanoma, the chance that any given dysplastic mole will become a melanoma is estimated at one in seven thousand.

A few melanomas don't make any stops along the tumor progression pathway: they become invasive in no time. One example of truncated evolution is the melanoma that seems to grow from a previously unblemished patch of skin. Another is the nodular melanoma that skips the flat radial growth phase.

When Should a Mole Be Removed?
People with many dysplastic nevi often have to have numerous biopsies. Happily, as is true of most colon polyps and breast lumps, most moles that are worrisome enough to be biopsied are not malignant.

So why not just take off all moles? Just as the prophylactic surgical removal of healthy breasts (that is, surgical removal of healthy tissue as a preventive measure) is a questionable way to prevent breast cancer, so the removal of all dysplastic or normal nevi is not recommended as a preventive to melanoma. Many people have too many moles for total removal to be practical; besides, melanoma may arise in apparently normal skin. Most important, though, most moles never act up.

Even though the wholesale removal of moles is overkill, sometimes you should have a mole removed. Here are some guidelines. If you have had melanoma and also have a solitary dysplastic nevus, have it taken off if it is easy and cosmetically acceptable to do so. If you have a changing or suspicious nevus, have it removed. If either you or your physician is concerned about a mole, especially one that appears to be changing, then it should be removed.

It is also important to know where your moles are and whether they are dysplastic or normal—and to watch them for changes. Richard Gallagher, head of Epidemiology for the British Columbia Cancer Agency, found from his numerous studies of moles and melanoma that many people pay no attention to their moles.

In one of his studies, interviewers asked melanoma patients if they recalled having had a mole in the place where their melanoma developed. Gallagher reports, "By and large, participants had no idea whether their melanoma originated from a pre-existing mole, or if they had any moles in corresponding sites of their bodies."

A study by members of the Melanoma Cooperative Group at New York University Medical Center followed a group of 357 patients with dysplastic nevi. Seventeen developed a total of eighteen melanomas, of which ten were invasive and eight were not invasive. Among a comparable set of patients, matched by sex and age, in the general population fewer than 1 would be expected to develop melanoma during that length of time. It is thus wise for people with dysplastic moles (or an abundance of ordinary moles) to keep a vigilant eye on them and have their physicians perform frequent skin exams to detect melanomas early in their evolution.[5]

Is Melanoma Hereditary? A misconception about melanoma (and cancer in general) is that it frequently runs in families and is probably caused by a mutant gene. In fact, only about one in ten patients with melanoma has a close family member who has also had melanoma.

Nevertheless, an important genetic connection exists. The National Cancer Institute and the University of Pennsylvania's Pigmented Lesion Group have been jointly studying twenty-three melanoma-prone families since 1976 to determine why melanoma clusters occur in families and how melanomas can be detected early. Studying these families has proved beneficial in gaining further knowledge about dysplastic nevi in general and in developing effective strategies for early detection and prevention for the 90 percent of the population without genes for melanoma susceptibility.

Doctors will strongly suspect that a family has a genetic tendency toward melanoma if a melanoma patient has two blood relatives—parents, siblings, or children—who have melanoma. Recently, several researchers have implicated a mutant gene on the ninth chromosome that regulates cell growth. In about a third of the families studied—families that did not display an unusual number of dysplastic nevi— the gene was broken. In fact, people who have the broken gene have a 50 percent chance of developing melanoma by the age of fifty. A few years ago, another gene was found to be responsible for producing melanoma in members of other melanoma-prone families who did have dysplastic nevi. Soon genetic testing for high susceptibility to melanoma will be possible, as it is for heightened susceptibility to breast and colon cancer.

Is a History of Skin Cancer a Risk Factor?

People who have had a more common kind of skin cancer, such as basal cell or squamous cell carcinoma, have an increased risk of getting melanoma. Not surprisingly, having had one melanoma also makes you more likely to develop a second.

If any of your family members have had melanoma or basal or squamous cell cancers, your risk for melanoma will rise, as well, probably because family members share several critical genes (for sun sensitivity, for example) and the same environment, rather than because they have a single mutant gene in common. As a child you may have spent a great deal of time vacationing with your family in sunny locations. Possibly you did not take preventive measures against sun exposure and thereby increased your risk of getting skin cancer. You may have inherited a type of skin that burns easily and never tans.

Among the families participating in the National Cancer Institute / Pigmented Lesion Group study, members with dysplastic nevi and one melanoma were found to be at very high risk, about two hundred times the average person's, of developing another melanoma. Some individuals have had more than ten separate melanomas. Dr. Allan Halpern found in a study of persons with no family history of melanoma that those with dysplastic nevi and one melanoma had a 30 percent chance of developing a second melanoma within ten years.[6]

In the United States, men and women get melanoma at about the same rates, yet in some countries, such as England and Scotland, women develop melanoma more frequently than men. Whether women in those countries spend more time in the sun than men do is unclear.

Regardless of how likely they are to get melanoma in the first place, women seem to survive longer than men once they have it. The natural assumption is that women's increased chance of survival is due to some hormonal or other protective factor. But epidemiologists also speculate that women are more health conscious and thus notice their melanomas earlier. Women may pay more attention to their appearance and as a consequence notice changes in their skin early on.[7]

Another explanation for their higher survival rate is that in women melanoma generally appears on the arms or legs, whereas the head and trunk are more common sites in men. And melanomas located on the extremities have a better prognosis.

Is Pregnancy a Risk Factor for Melanoma?

Young women often become pregnant and sometimes get melanoma. The concurrence of the two events is emotionally charged, and it is easy to believe that they are causally related. One study suggests that melanomas are thicker in pregnant women than in non-pregnant women.[8] It is also known that moles—and the skin (for instance, of the cheeks, nipples, and the line between the navel and the pubis) tend to darken during pregnancy. Still, despite a certain amount of anecdotal evidence, any connection between pregnancy and melanoma is probably coincidental.

Most physicians will advise women not to get pregnant for at least two to three years after a diagnosis of melanoma, because the risk of recurrence is highest during this time. Women may not want to cope simultaneously with the psychological and physical stresses of caring for a young child and with the prospect of such a recurrence.

Will Taking Oral Contraceptives or Undergoing Hormone Replacement Therapy Increase a Woman's Risk?

Elizabeth Holly, professor of epidemiology and biostatistics at the School of Medicine, University of California at San Francisco, has pioneered studies on hormones affecting the growth of melanoma. In a 1994 study (published in *Cancer Epidemiology, Biomarkers and Prevention*) Dr. Holly examined 452 women aged twenty-five to fifty-nine who had been diagnosed with superficial spreading melanoma. A control group of more than 900 women of the same age group who did not have melanoma provided the comparison.[9]

She studied all the women to determine whether they were at increased risk for developing melanoma after they had had menopausal hormone replacement therapy or used birth control pills. Holly says she found only a "a hint of something going on hormonally that may have influenced the development of melanoma." Although she detected a statistically insignificant increase in the incidence of melanoma among all the women treated with hormones, she concluded that the benefits of hormone replacement therapy in preventing osteoporosis and heart disease and in mitigating the symptoms of menopause should outweigh the concern about the possible increased risk of melanoma. In addition, there is no reason to advise women who have had melanoma to avoid taking oral contraceptives.[10] A 1993 study conducted in Germany corroborated Holly's findings. It revealed that neither hormones produced during pregnancy nor oral contraceptives had an effect on melanoma patients' prognosis.[11] The results of a large pooled analysis in which Dr. Holly and her colleagues will examine all studies pertaining to hormone use and melanoma will be available shortly.

Does It Matter Where a Person Lives?

Living close to the equator is associated with a higher incidence of melanoma among Caucasians. White residents of Queensland, Australia, have the highest rate in the world: forty melanoma patients per hundred thousand people. Sunny areas of the United States also have high rates of melanoma. Southern Arizona, for example, has an incidence of twenty-six per hundred thousand.

An interesting exception to this pattern is that rates of melanoma in northern Europe (for example, Sweden and Norway) are generally higher than in southern Europe (for example, France and Italy), even after differences in skin type have been taken into account. Epidemiologists suggest that the sun-seeking behavior of northern Europeans may account for the phenomenon. Because their long, dark winters leave them sun-starved, when it *is* sunny they throw caution (and clothing) to the wind.

Writing this chapter forced me to re-evaluate why a melanoma formed on my leg. Although I am a health-conscious person, I had no idea how closely I conformed to the profile of a person at high risk for melanoma.

My fair skin is freckled and burns easily. Although I do not think of myself as a sun worshiper, during the first eight years of my life I lived in southern Arizona and was an avid swimmer. I used baby oil in place of suntan lotion. In addition to that intense sun exposure in childhood, I tanned my legs with a sunlamp in high school.

I have no family history of melanoma, but some of my sisters have had basal cell skin cancers. I had a funny-looking mole where the melanoma formed, on the back of my leg; and while writing this book, I also developed squamous cell cancer.

Because it had entered the vertical growth phase when it was found, my melanoma was a threat. I am still amazed that I found it when I did. It was located on an area of my body that could have gone unnoticed for some time, especially given my frantic pace of life. In hindsight, I would have preferred to know that I was at risk. I wonder now whether I could have avoided melanoma entirely, had my physician talked to me about examining my skin and had my parents known to shield me from overexposure.

4 | Finding Early Melanoma

The lifetime risk of getting melanoma was 1 in 250 in 1980; by the year 2000 it will be 1 in 75 (American Cancer Society pamphlet, 1994). Melanoma has long had the reputation of being deadly, and in the 1930s, when the mortality rate stood at 75 percent, it was. The current death rate from melanoma has dropped to under 15 percent, according to the same American Cancer Society publication. The statistic is proof that identification of early melanoma allows remarkably effective therapy.

Fortunately, melanoma is visible to the naked eye. It is pigmented and begins in the top layer of the skin. These features differentiate melanoma from the other potentially serious cancers and make it easier to spot and treat early. Melanoma is different from many other cancers in a second respect: we know the carcinogen. Sunlight is a major trigger for the changes in melanocytes that can later result in melanoma.

Still, although they are easy to recognize early on, many melanomas go unnoticed until the later stages, when they are less likely to be curable. Doctors are a long way from being able to treat advanced-stage melanoma with gene manipulation and vaccination; such techniques still represent a medical frontier. (See Chapter 6.) Along with prevention, early detection is still the best line of defense and should be made a top priority in the battle against melanoma. It is important to teach the public, primary health care providers, and body care practitioners how to recognize incipient melanoma. Early detection will translate into a savings in lives, and at a remarkably low cost.

When Is Melanoma Curable? Melanoma is always curable when completely removed before it develops the capacity to spread. In March 1992, Dr. Guerry and his colleagues found, after following six hundred patients over the course of thirteen years, that the one-third of the invasive melanomas caught in the radial growth phase did not metastasize (spread) to the rest of the body. The study also revealed that an early melanoma lesion takes a few years on average to advance to the vertical growth phase, when it might metastasize.[1] Thus, ample opportunity usually exists for early detection. Nevertheless, some early melanomas don't give you that latitude but metastasize more rapidly. So it's important not to put off having your doctor check out any suspicious signs you may notice.

As mentioned in Chapter 2, the earliest step is melanoma in situ (in its place of origin)—confined to the epidermis. Pathologist Wallace Clark spoke of the "radial growth phase" because early melanoma appears as an irregular circular blotch on the skin that gradually expands along the radii of an imperfect circle. The next step in early melanoma is the invasive radial growth phase, called invasive because the melanoma extends into the dermis from the epidermis. (See Figure 21.) Melanomas treated at either of these steps are apparently 100 percent curable. The next step is the vertical growth phase, in which a part of the melanoma often starts to elevate (become dome-shaped) as it grows in and through the underlying dermis. Even at this later stage, the overall cure rate is 70 percent. Still, the sooner melanoma is caught, the better: small melanomas in the vertical growth phase are more likely to be cured than larger ones.

How Do I Find Early Melanoma?

Regular skin examination is crucial to finding early melanoma at its most curable stage, so you should set up a schedule of self-examinations. (See Figure 22 for instructions and illustrations on how to do a self-exam.)

If you have a personal or family history of melanoma or dysplastic nevi, check yourself monthly and have a dermatologist or a physician who is knowledgeable about melanoma check you frequently, too. The frequency of the doctor's exams should be based on the level of risk. For patients at very high risk, as many as four visits per year may be recommended. Self-examination is crucial as a supplement to professional follow-up. Patients have demonstrated that they can spot a significant skin lesion just as readily as a physician can if they are educated properly. As Berwick and others reported in the *Journal of the National Cancer Institute* in 1996, people who regularly check themselves for suspicious skin changes are 44 percent less likely to die

Figure 22. Skin Examination: How to Do It

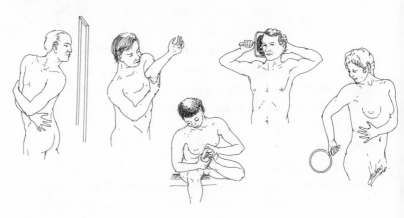

of melanoma than those who do not check.[2] If you are at higher than average risk, you should examine your skin monthly. Mark the date on the calendar. For women, a good way to remember to do the self-exam is to tie it in with their breast exam. If you are at average to low risk for melanoma, you can certainly do skin self-exams less frequently, every six months or annually. A partner can help you see such hard-to-examine areas as your back and scalp.

Skin Examination: How to Do It, What to Look For

Start your skin examination in a brightly lighted room. You'll need a hand-held flashlight, a full-length mirror, a hand mirror, and two chairs or stools.

1. With your back turned to the full-length mirror, inspect the back of your neck and shoulders. Check your face in the

mirror, concentrating on your lips, mouth, and ears (front
and back).

2. Check your hands by examining the palms and backs; look
   between the fingers and under the fingernails. Continue up
   the wrists to examine both the front and back of your fore-
   arms. Scan all sides of your upper arms—don't forget to look
   at underarms too.

3. Sit down, prop each leg in turn on the other stool or chair.
   Check the front and sides of both legs, thigh to shin: the an-
   kles, the tops of the feet, between the toes, and under the
   toenails. Examine the heels and the soles of the feet.

4. Using a hand-held mirror, focus on the neck, chest, and
   torso. Women should check the undersides of the breasts,
   the upper back, and any part of the upper arms not viewed
   in step 2.

5. Using both mirrors, scan your lower back and buttocks and
   the backs of both legs.

As was discussed extensively in Chapter 3, normal moles
are small, flat or dome-shaped skin blemishes or growths,
whereas dysplastic nevi are larger, unusual-looking moles
that can be warning signs for an increased risk of getting
malignant melanoma. Early melanoma can look like an irregular, inflamed, or spreading flat mole. To help people
know and recognize the look of early melanoma, the
mnemonic the "ABCDE's" of melanoma was coined.

- *Asymmetry:* The growth has an irregular shape: one half of the
  pigmented spot doesn't look like the other half.
- *Border irregularity:* The border is irregular or notched, not
  smooth like the round or oval outline of a normal mole.
- *Color variation:* normal moles are usually one color, whereas
  a melanoma may be different hues of tan, brown, dark
  brown, blue, pink, black, or even white.
- *Diameter:* A pigmented spot that is larger than six millimeters

or one that is clearly growing may be a problem. Melanomas grow to become larger than ordinary moles: a pigmented spot with a diameter bigger than half a centimeter (or a quarter of an inch) should be scrutinized. Any pigmented spot with a diameter of about a centimeter (three-eighths of an inch) requires evaluation.

- *Elevation:* Some early melanomas are slightly elevated throughout, like a little mesa. Any pigmented lesion that quickly elevates throughout or develops a bump should be checked right away.

The only drawback of the ABCDE's is that they do not emphasize the dynamic quality of many melanomas, that is their tendency to change noticeably over weeks or months. *Change* is the key word and one of the American Cancer Society's Seven Warning Signs of Cancer: "a change in a wart or mole." If you notice a color change, particularly some darkening within a pigmented spot, or an enlargement of a previously stable mole or the appearance of a new pigmented spot of about half a centimeter in diameter—particularly if you are twenty-five or older—have a dermatologist or physician familiar with melanoma check it out. And don't be afraid or embarrassed to see someone about the skin change.

Professional Skin Examinations   Don't expect your family doctor to perform a skin examination unless you have specifically requested it. And do request it! Many general practitioners don't make skin exams a normal part of a routine physical, nor do they teach self-examination techniques. Because little time is spent in medical school teaching the technique of skin examination, few practitioners are sufficiently aware of its importance.

Doctors today are overwhelmed already by the number of screening tests they have been told they should perform.

If you are at high risk for melanoma, your first check-up should include a complete skin examination, risk assessment, education about the warning signs of melanoma and the best way to protect yourself and your family from overexposure to the sun. A few people should have baseline photographs of their skin taken for purposes of comparison on subsequent visits. Skin may change more during hormonal fluctuations, so the skin should be checked more frequently during pregnancy.

If you are still worried about something on your skin and your medical practitioner doesn't satisfy your concern, seek another opinion, preferably from a dermatologist. Melanomas can be tricky to diagnose. It's your body, and you should trust your intuition if you think something is wrong. Don't wait for potentially more serious symptoms or signs to arise, such as a pigmented spot with lumpiness, crusting, oozing, bleeding, or ulceration.

Two other features of melanoma are also worth mentioning. Some melanomas look ugly and may give rise to comment. If someone says to you, "What's that? You should get that taken care of!" do it. Some melanomas, and of course a lot of other things, itch or sting persistently. Any pigmented lesion that does should be checked.

Where Do Melanomas Most Often Appear?

Melanomas most commonly appear on the backs of people of both sexes, the chests and abdomens of men, and the legs of women. A 1995 study found the most common melanoma site for women to be legs, unless the woman had a dysplastic nevus, in which case the melanoma was more likely to appear on the trunk.[3] Surprisingly, melanomas can also occasionally arise in places unexposed to sun, such as the underarms, buttocks, or groin or on or under the breasts in women. The sun may act systemically as well as directly on the body; or melanoma may have other causes besides intense sunlight.

Unfortunately, many people don't realize that something growing on the outside of their body is potentially lethal. Others, by contrast, worry so much about a spot that they go into denial and don't attempt to find out what is wrong. Studies show that people don't get an early melanoma checked and treated because it grows slowly and doesn't "stick out," or they haven't experienced any particularly alarming or annoying symptoms, such as the bleeding or ulceration that usually occurs after the melanoma has progressed to a later stage.

A ten-year study at the Pigmented Lesion Clinic of patients with superficial spreading melanoma found that people waited an average of nine months to get a lesion checked. A long lag time between diagnosis and treatment can result in a less favorable prognosis. In the same study it was reported that in some cases physicians were responsible for the delay, because they didn't recognize the melanoma for what it was or didn't adequately examine the skin.[4] Both these failures can be blamed on insufficient medical and public health education.

Warning Others   Once you become knowledgeable about the "look" of melanoma, you may find yourself facing the dilemma of spotting something that could be melanoma on strangers and not knowing how to approach them. Dr. Guerry says he doesn't hesitate to point out suspicious lesions to people he doesn't know. Of course he can explain that he is a doctor and knows what he is talking about.

Although I had no medical credentials to fall back on, I did stick my neck out and speak to a young woman in an exercise class I was taking. She had a very obvious melanoma on her upper arm—I could see it from across the room. I found myself in the awkward position of needing to urge her to get to the doctor quickly without frightening her. When I told her my suspicion, she put me off, saying that she would wait until her annual gynecological exam. Knowing the consequences of late detection, I decided to pursue the matter. I talked to a mutual friend, who called the woman's husband. He applied additional pressure, and a month later, she had her arm checked by a dermatologist. It was melanoma—an early one. Although you may naturally hesitate to approach someone about so personal a matter, you may well save that person's life by speaking up.

In 1992 Howard Koh, director of cancer prevention and control at the Boston University School of Medicine, did a study of 216 melanoma cases to determine who most often found melanoma. The patients themselves had found 53 percent of the lesions. In 26 percent of the cases, medical care providers (of whom only 3 percent were dermatologists) discovered the melanoma. Family members found 17 percent and others, 4 percent.[5]

Women were the champion melanoma spotters in this study—the most likely to discover their own melanomas—regardless of the anatomical site of the lesion—and their partners', whereas men rarely were responsible for finding their own or their partners' melanomas. Among women, for instance, 71 percent located the lesions on their own backs. That nearly 26 percent of men did not see their own back lesions easily underlines the potential utility of performing skin examinations with a partner's assistance.[6]

Koh's study has important implications for preventive education; men should be specially targeted in public health campaigns because they may be less likely to have themselves checked by a doctor early on. (See Chapter 8.)

Another important outcome of the study was the inference that dermatologists play a small role in melanoma *detection* (although they play a large role in therapy and follow-up). Especially in these days of managed care, when concerns about cost containment make it increasingly difficult for patients to see specialists, it is important for other medical professionals who examine the patients more frequently—nurses, nurse-midwives, paramedics, family practitioners, pediatricians, obstetricians and gynecologists, and physical therapists—to be trained to recognize melanoma. Also, nonmedical professionals who tend to people's health and personal care—hairdressers, massage therapists, lifeguards, and health club personnel, among others—can play an important role in screening.

Are There Any Free Screening Programs for Melanoma? Since 1985, the American Academy of Dermatology (AAD) has operated a free screening program; as of this writing, 750,000 people have been screened. Call the AAD to find out about a program in your area. (See Appendix B.) Dr. Allan Halpern, who co-directed the Pigmented Lesion Group and now directs the AAD's prevention program, says that "50 percent of those screened would not have seen a doctor for a skin examination without the free program, and 35 percent gave a history of a changing mole, the most sensitive risk factor for the presence of melanoma."[7]

By contrast with Pap smear screening, which is forty years old, skin cancer screening is still in its infancy. (It has been practiced for only about twenty years.) Many in the medical profession feel that screenings are not cost-effective, and they worry that they will be liable to malpractice suits if skin cancer is missed. Although no randomized trial has been done to see how many lives skin cancer screening saves, a recent encounter I had with a melanoma patient at a support group is indicative of the effectiveness of screening. This woman had a mole checked at a skin cancer screening held at her place of employment. She is certain that if that screening had not been offered, she would be dealing with something much more serious now, because she would not have had it checked otherwise. Thanks to screening, the melanoma was detected in its early stages, and she was directed to a dermatologist.

Recent evaluation of nationwide screening in the AAD's programs between 1989 and 1992 revealed that 90 percent of all melanomas detected were less than 1.5 millimeters thick. Of those persons with a screening diagnosis who attended the 1992–93 programs, all but 4 of the 261 confirmed melanomas were relatively early disease.[8]

Targeting Those at Risk In Chapter 3 we saw who is at higher than average risk for melanoma (those with fair skin that freckles and burns easily, those with a personal or family history of melanoma or nonmelanoma skin cancers, and those with many ordinary moles or any dysplastic moles). But how do you reach these people and convince them to get their skin checked? As Howard Koh puts it, "What happens if you hold a party and the wrong people show up?" Dr. Guerry stresses that "how to target, reach, and motivate the segment of the population at high risk of getting melanoma is an important research question." "The answer," he says "will have important elements of self-assessment (of sun sensitivity and exposure, of family history) and self-examination (for sun damage, freckling, many moles, dysplastic moles, any spots suspicious for melanoma)." Dr. Richard Sagebiel, director of the University of California at San Francisco / Mount Zion Melanoma Center, remarks: "The best way to screen the population at large would be to look at the skin of white people employed in an upscale office building." A novel but effective approach in many areas is to set up a tent on the local beach and invite people in their bathing attire for screening.

Having found it comfortable and not unduly inconvenient, most people who have been to a screening recommend it to friends and relatives. According to Dr. Koh, "One of the best features of screening is that it offers an educational moment."[9] The physician has the opportunity to explain skin cancer prevention while examining the patient.

5 If You Have Melanoma

According to the American Cancer Society, the incidence of melanoma among whites doubled between 1973 and 1991 and is increasing faster than that of any other type of cancer.[1] It is natural for people to vacillate between compulsion and complacency when it comes to taking care of their bodies. Sometimes when they find something wrong, they put off getting it checked because they think it's probably nothing; or they're so worried that it might be something serious, like cancer, that they avoid seeking medical attention altogether.

When you spot something suspicious growing on your skin, don't procrastinate. Have it checked. Melanoma usually doesn't grow so rapidly that a suspicious growth should be cause for panic, but a biopsy needs to be done expeditiously. Your doctor can't treat an unknown. Dr. Guerry points out that more often than not, a pigmented spot is *not* melanoma: "Many benign pigmented lesions masquerade as melanoma."

If you are in a health maintenance organization, as many Americans are, you are probably required to see your primary care physician first for any problems. If your primary care physician is judicious, and skilled, by all means entrust him or her with figuring out what the spot is. As pointed out before, it is a good idea to ask your doctor to examine your skin thoroughly early on and at appropriate intervals thereafter.

If your doctor is concerned about the lesion you point out, he or she may want to biopsy it or might refer you to a dermatologist or a surgeon for further checks and a biopsy. If your doctor says to watch the skin lesion and come back in six months, insist that it be checked sooner—say, in a month or two—or ask for a referral to a dermatologist. You may run into some resistance, now that many health plans restrict the number of referrals to specialists, so be persistent.

What Is the Best Biopsy Procedure? As a general rule, excisional biopsies are the best, because they are designed to remove the entire lesion. The pathologist needs to look at a representative specimen to make the diagnosis of melanoma and to determine the features that predict its behavior.

Excisional biopsies are usually relatively painless. After a local anesthetic is administered, the suspicious spot and a small margin around it are removed, and a few stitches are taken to close the wound. You can resume most activities a few days later.

In certain circumstances other types of biopsies may be appropriate. If the lesion is small and located in a cosmetically sensitive area, such as your face, a deep shave biopsy may be performed. In this procedure, after a local anesthetic is injected, the spot is shaved off with a razor blade. A punch biopsy or an incisional biopsy may sometimes be used in the case of a large lesion. In the first technique, the most alarming part of the lesion is "punched out" with a cookie cutter–like instrument. In the second, a small portion of the spot is cut out with a scalpel. With either method, disturbance to the appearance of the face, for example, is minimal.

One of the myths about melanoma is that a biopsy will stir up the melanoma cells and cause them to infiltrate the body. No evidence indicates that this will happen. The concern is that a shave biopsy may make it difficult to determine the extent to which melanoma has penetrated the skin, and consequently to determine its stage accurately.

What Should I Ask?   Here are some questions to ask and answers to look for when you see a doctor about a suspicious skin growth.

1. What do you think this thing is? (Make sure your concern over it is taken seriously.) Most often the diagnosis will be something like seborrheic keratosis (which is a benign lesion) or an ordinary mole.

2. (If the doctor says that no biopsy is necessary) Are you sure this lesion is benign? Do you think it's sufficient simply to keep an eye on the lesion? Ascertain the doctor's degree of comfort with the diagnosis. If the doctor dismisses the growth as nothing worrisome, yet you have a gut feeling that it needs to be checked further, get it done.

3. (If a biopsy is to be done) Do you plan to do an excisional biopsy? If not, why not?

4. When will the results of the biopsy be available? A week is usually enough time to make a determination.

What Is a Pathology Report?   After the biopsy is completed, the specimen is
sent to a pathologist, a specially trained physician who interprets the nature of your lesion by examining the biopsy
specimen under a microscope. The pathologist's role in
proper diagnosis of a pigmented spot is critical: he or she
makes the determination whether it is benign, indeterminate, or malignant and, if it is malignant, what its attributes
are. Your doctor takes this information into account in recommending a treatment. That's why it is important to make
sure that your biopsy is interpreted by a skilled pathologist.

Your doctor will receive the pathologist's report. If the
report describes the lesion as suspicious or hard to interpret, you should request that the specimen be reviewed by
a dermatopathologist—a specialist in the pathology of the
skin—or by a pathologist specializing in melanoma. Such
specialized pathologists are often associated with teaching
hospitals. Be sure to ask for a copy of your pathology report,
even if you don't want to read it. When you ask for it, your
physician or the office staff may react with puzzlement. Simply explain that you like to keep accurate medical records for
future reference.

As with any cancer, accurate interpretation of the pathology is crucial in determining proper treatment. The attributes discussed in the pathology report, together with
your physical examination, will usually provide an indication
of what surgery is needed, whether you require additional
tests and therapy, and what the outcome of the disease is
likely to be. The biopsy report will contain valuable information that you will need later, and if you require a second

doctor's opinion, it will speed things up to have the pathology report on hand. Most physicians will also wish to have the glass pathology slides available for review by an expert before offering a second opinion.

Even if you are content with your doctor's diagnosis and treatment plan, it may be a good idea to get a second opinion. Opinions on treatment and prognosis of melanoma may differ even when doctors agree on the pathology results. Especially in high-risk situations, going the extra mile is worth the trouble even if you are worn out by worry.

Two of the important characteristics of your melanoma described in the pathology report are its biological growth phase and the likelihood of spreading (or metastasis). In 1969 Dr. Wallace Clark was one of the first to distinguish between melanomas that apparently could not spread beyond their site of origin (and thus were still in the radial growth phase—see Chapter 4) and melanomas that had become lumpy (that is, established the vertical growth phase) and had some chance of spreading to other parts of the body.

He also categorized melanomas by level (later to be termed Clark level) to designate which layer of the skin they had penetrated to. All level I and many level II melanomas are radial growth phase melanomas; the deeper-level melanomas—III, IV, and V—routinely enter the vertical growth phase. The higher the Clark level, the greater the probability that the cancer will spread. (See Figure 23.)

In the early 1970s, Dr. Alexander Breslow of George Washington University Medical School found that it was simpler and more accurate to base the prognosis on the

Figure 23. Levels and Thickness of Melanomas

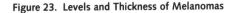

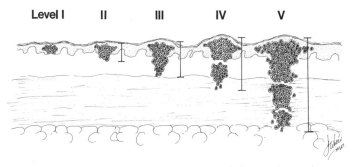

Levels describe the anatomical layer of the skin into which the melanoma has penetrated. All level I and most level II melanomas are pure radial growth phase melanomas and do not metastasize. The brackets show how thickness is measured.

pathologist's measurement (in millimeters) of the thickness of a melanoma that had penetrated below the epidermis than to base the prognosis on the level of melanoma.

Probably the most accurate way to predict how patients will do is to distinguish between radial growth phase melanomas (which have essentially no likelihood of recurrence) and vertical growth phase melanomas. Further examination of vertical growth phase melanomas allows the physician to better estimate the chance of cure.

Drs. Clark and his associates at the Pigmented Lesion Group pulled together these predictive attributes of melanomas and patients in their "Model Predicting Survival in Stage I Melanoma Based on Tumor Progression." The report presented a table of six attributes (see items 3–8 in the list that follows), which, taken together, can predict survival more accurately than tumor thickness alone can.[2]

Dr. Lynn Schuchter, a member of the Pigmented Lesion Group at the University of Pennsylvania hospital, recently devised a simplified way of predicting outcome in melanoma patients. She first examined one hundred pathology reports from different pathologists. Only half the reports mentioned either the thickness of the melanoma or the level of invasion. None of the reports mentioned whether the cancer was still entirely in the radial growth phase. After following 488 patients at the Pigmented Lesion Clinic for 13.5 years, Dr. Schuchter found four independent factors that pathologists and clinicians anywhere could ascertain about patients and their tumor: the patient's age and sex and the melanoma's thickness and location. Basing the prognosis on these attributes rather than just thickness reduced by 50 percent the margin of error in predicting survival.[3]

Alternative predictive models now available to clinicians help pinpoint attributes such as ulceration of the tumor. Now that pathologists are reporting more information for use in these improved models, physicians are better equipped to counsel their patients on options for therapy.

It is always useful to have your doctor translate your pathology report. Dr. Clark's pathology report for me in 1989 is reproduced here as an example. (See Figure 24.) This report touched on most of the variables discussed in the 1989 study mentioned earlier and made a prediction about the chances of survival. Your report may look different—there is as yet no standardized pathology report—but most will show some of the same factors. It would be a mistake for doctors to oversimplify by relying on a single pathology variable as an accurate prediction of how you will do.

Figure 24. Pathology Report of C. Poole

UNIVERSITY of PENNSYLVANIA

Wallace H. Clark, Jr., M.D.
Department of Dermatology
250 Medical Education Building
30th and Hamilton Walk
Philadelphia, PA 19104-6013
215-898-3231

CP110146
No charge

18 January 1989

Chanchal Khanna, MD
Department of Pathology
Doylestown Hospital
595 West State Street
US Routes 202 & 611 Bypass
Doylestown, PA 18901

RE: POOLE, Catherine
WHC 2260
Your 89-66

Dear Doctor Khanna:

The material accessioned under the above name and numbers shows a compound nevus with some atypia. As such, this may be regarded as dysplastic. Superimposed upon this there is some upward growth of melanocytes in a single area, associated with ulceration, where atypical cells can extend into the reticular dermis. There are mitotic figures associated with the ulceration but they are also present away from this.

DIAGNOSIS: MALIGNANT MELANOMA

Type:	Superficial spreading type
Growth Phase:	Radial growth phase present
	Vertical growth phase present
Mitotic Count:	1/mm^2
Tumor Infiltrating Lymphocytes:	Absent
Greatest Thickness:	0.75mm
Level of Invasion:	Level IV
Site:	Calf
Sex:	Female
Regression:	Absent
Precursor Lesion:	Compound nevus with melanocytic
	dysplasia of the type seen in the
	dysplastic nevus syndrome

RISK FACTORS: The tumor has entered the vertical growth phase but the potential for metastasis is not great. In our data base,

---

UNIVERSITY of PENNSYLVANIA

WHC 2260

Wallace H. Clark, Jr., M.D.
Department of Dermatology
250 Medical Education Building
30th and Hamilton Walk
Philadelphia, PA 19104-6013
215-898-3231

–Page 2 –

cases with similar attributes have a probability of survival at 8 years of .95 with a 95% confidence interval that extends from .88 to .98.

Thank you for referring this material. Best regards.

Sincerely yours,

Wallace H Clark, Jr, MD
WHC:cpb

Here is an explanation of the terms in my pathology report:

1. *Type:* description of the particular variety of growth you have—superficial spreading melanoma, lentigo maligna melanoma, nodular melanoma, and so on. The superficial spreading type is the most common. (See Chapter 2 for an explanation of the different types of melanoma.)

2. *Growth phase:* designation that shows whether the melanoma has reached the step where it can grow as a lump below the epidermis. In the radial growth phase, as we have seen, it is unlikely that the cancer has begun to metastasize. By the vertical growth phase, there is at least some chance that the disease has spread elsewhere in the body.

3. *Mitotic count:* measure of how many cells are dividing below the epidermis. Only in the vertical growth phase do cells divide in the dermis. The higher the mitotic count, the more likely the tumor is to spread.

4. *Tumor-infiltrating lymphocytes:* immune system cells (lymphocytes) whose presence in the vertical growth phase are a positive sign. Presumably, lymphocytes show that the immune system has recognized the tumor and is attacking it.

5. *Greatest thickness:* the Breslow thickness. A measurement of less than a millimeter is considered thin—and means a favorable prognosis.

6. *Site:* location of the melanoma. Patients with a vertical growth phase melanoma located on an extremity have a relatively favorable prognosis, unless the lesion appears on the palms, on the soles of the feet, or under the nails.

7. *Sex:* gender of the melanoma patient. For unexplained reasons, women have a better prognosis than men.

8. *Regression:* Attribute that may be either absent or present in the radial growth phase (which is adjacent to the vertical growth phase). Regression is evidence of destruction (probably by immune factors) of some of the melanoma cells in

the radial growth phase. Immunologically mediated regression of this sort is a weakly negative factor.

9. *Level of invasion:* the Clark level. Mine was a level IV tumor—that is, the melanoma had penetrated to just above the fatty layer of the skin.

10. *Precursor lesion:* Evidence of a pre-existing ordinary, dysplastic, or congenital mole from which the melanoma might have developed. My melanoma came from a dysplastic nevus. Although dysplastic nevi are the most common precursors, common moles and congenital moles may also be culprits. For many melanomas no evidence of a precursor shows up.

Risk Factors "The tumor has entered the vertical growth phase but the potential for metastasis is not great. In our data base, cases with similar attributes have a probability of survival at 8 years .95 with 95% confidence interval that extends from .88 to .98."

This means that in a population of patients who have melanomas with these attributes, 95 percent (with a range of between 88 and 98 percent) can expect to be cured by appropriate surgical removal of their melanoma.

According to Dr. Guerry, my chance of survival then was very good (and now is nearly perfect because so much time has elapsed), but for about 5 percent of people, melanomas like mine are fatal, a "sobering . . . reminder of the importance of follow-up to find treatable recurrences early and of the need for additional therapy beyond surgery in some people."

Questions to Ask Your Doctor About the Pathology Report

1. Who will read the pathology? An expert dermatopathologist should probably be on hand if the lesion is difficult to identify or characterize.

2. Will the doctor be available to discuss the pathology with me? The nurse may telephone you if the biopsy shows that the growth is trivial (a seborrheic keratosis or an ordinary mole), but if it is more serious (say, a nonmelanoma dysplastic mole, or melanoma), you should be able to consult personally with your physician.

3. What exactly does this pathology mean? If it is melanoma, how do its attributes affect my prognosis?

4. What do you recommend as the next course of action?

What Are the Stages of Melanoma?

After looking at the pathology report, physicians assign a "stage" to cancer as a means to classify their patients according to their chances of being cured, and to guide their choice of treatment. In general, doctors integrate information on the primary tumor with data on the presence and location of metastases to arrive at the stage. For instance:

- Stage I: The tumor is up to 1.5 millimeters thick; no evidence of nearby skin or lymph node involvement or of distant metastasis. The five-year survival rate is about 95 percent.

- Stage II: The primary tumor is more than 1.5 millimeters thick; no evidence of spread. The five-year survival rate is about 80 percent. Note that the outcome for patients with Stage I and II disease can be more accurately forecast with the predictive models described earlier.

- Stage III: Melanoma has spread into the lymph glands (nodes) near the primary tumor. (The regional nodes for a melanoma on the right forearm, for example, are in the right armpit.) The five-year survival rate is about 50 percent.
- Stage IV: Colonies of melanoma cells are evident beyond the regional nodes (for example, in the distant skin or nodes or in the organs in the body). The five-year survival rate is about 10 percent.

Remember that these methods of predicting outcomes, although useful in judging how a group of people will do, are often remarkably inadequate in foretelling your particular future.

What Are Lymph Nodes? The body's lymphatic system comprises lymph (which is a fluid), lymph vessels, and lymph nodes. Lymph carries lymphocytes and other cells of the immune system, together with invading bacteria and waste products, through the tissues. Lymph is transported through lymph vessels, the microscopic tubes that carry it into the nodes. Lymph nodes are little glands that contain millions of immune system cells. Clusters of lymph nodes are located in strategic places throughout the body. Lymph nodes are an important component of the immune system—the place where immune cells, primarily lymphocytes, are marshaled to fight invaders. Thus, the lymph nodes in your neck may swell when your body is trying to fight off an upper respiratory tract infection. Melanoma cells also may travel through lymph vessels into lymph nodes and start reproducing inside them.

If melanoma has spread to your lymph nodes, the disease takes on a different character. Lymph node involvement generally overshadows the pathology of the primary lesion in significance. Melanoma has declared itself as an actual rather than a potential invader. It is exploiting the lymphatic system to colonize new territory.

Even once melanoma has successfully penetrated the body to reach nearby lymph nodes, the cure rate is considerable. On average, 40 to 50 percent of those with regional node involvement are cured. (The overall range is 15 to 70 percent, depending on the number of lymph nodes involved and other factors.)

If your physician feels an enlarged regional lymph node either on your first visit or in follow-up, you will probably be advised to have a biopsy (with a needle or a scalpel) of the node. If melanoma is found, a node dissection may be warranted.

What Is a Lymph Node Dissection?   If melanoma is found in a regional node but nowhere else, you will be advised to have a node dissection—that is, to have the majority of the nodes in that region (for example, the armpit or the groin) surgically removed. (Don't worry; you have plenty of other lymph nodes to take up the slack.)

Some people whose lymph nodes are obviously enlarged by a colony of melanoma cells can be cured by surgery; a long-standing question has been whether patients whose nodes are not enlarged (but who may be harboring

microscopic colonies) might likewise benefit from the removal of regional nodes.

Recent research indicates that some patients clearly do
not gain anything from elective or prophylactic node dissection at the site of the primary tumor around the time of surgery. These patients' melanoma is unlikely to metastasize,
to the nodes or elsewhere. Patients with pure radial growth
phase melanomas or with "thin" lesions (less than a millimeter thick) fall into this category.[4]

Patients in whom colonies of melanoma have probably
already been established beyond the regional nodes, such
as those whose melanomas are more than four millimeters
thick, will not benefit from a dissection either. What about
people with melanomas of intermediate thickness? Couldn't
the patients (still the minority) who have microscopic colonies in their nodes benefit from node removal before the
colonies adapt and propagate elsewhere? This issue is still
unresolved. A recent large study of almost 750 patients indicates that among patients under sixty years old, an additional 10 percent with a tumor one to two millimeters thick
may survive if they have an elective node dissection. Such
patients' five-year survival rate is 96 percent, as opposed to
86 percent for those who wait to have nodes removed when
and if they become swollen with melanoma.[5]

What Is Lymphoscintigraphy? It is often straightforward
enough to figure out what
lymph node group a melanoma might travel to. Melanomas of the leg colonize the nodes in the crease of the groin

(inguinal nodes), and arm melanomas wind up in the armpit (axillary nodes). In other areas, the back for example, the
melanoma cells' destination isn't so obvious. A melanoma of
the skin over the right shoulder blade might wind up in the
left armpit or the right groin. To find the general destination
of such melanomas, physicians have started using a technique called lymphoscintigraphy. It involves injecting a
small amount of radioactive material around the site of a
primary melanoma and then scanning different areas—the
armpits and groin, for example—to see which one or ones
"light up."

What Is Sentinel Lymph Node Biopsy?

A technique called sentinel
lymph node biopsy has been
designed to determine whether
the lymph node that would potentially receive colonies of
cells from the primary melanoma has actually done so. The
information about the melanoma's lymph node drainage
gleaned from lymphoscintigraphy is refined to identify the
"sentinel lymph node"—the first lymph node to receive
melanoma colonies—and to draw a sample from it. The sentinel node is identified by injecting a radioactive solution or
a blue-colored dye or both into the spot where the primary
melanoma is (or was), but this procedure must be carried
out prior to re-excision of the primary melanoma site. After
waiting half an hour or so for the dye to travel through the
lymph vessels to the node, the surgeon identifies the lymph
node group with a radioactivity probe and, with a small incision, removes it for a pathology examination. If after a few
days the node is found not to contain melanoma, then the

adjacent nodes are very unlikely to be involved and no further surgery is necessary. If the sentinel node does reveal melanoma, however, the adjacent nodes are removed in what is called a completion node dissection, because the chance is significant that they are involved as well.

What Are the Pros and Cons of These Techniques?

This new way of determining the stage of a melanoma, lymph node mapping and sentinel node harvesting, promises to give both patient and doctor more information more efficiently. Unless the nodes are involved, the patient is spared all but the small incision to check the sentinel node. Also, the removal of nodes containing melanoma may in itself increase the chance of cure. If the doctor determines that the lymph nodes are involved, the patient may be offered nonsurgical adjuvant therapy that will increase the chance of survival.

The downside is that with the advent of lymph node mapping and sentinel lymph node harvesting, the decision about what to do at this stage when the patient's regional lymph nodes appear normal has become more difficult. Some melanoma specialists speculate that lymph node mapping and sentinel node harvesting will become a necessity for all patients whose melanomas show a likelihood of metastasizing. Other specialists believe that the best course is to watch and wait. Mapping and harvesting remains an experimental approach. Dr. Guerry urges patients to participate in the experimental trials of the effectiveness of this technique but tells people who cannot that no one has yet proven the value of sentinel node biopsy in saving lives.

Here are some questions you should ask your doctor about regional lymph node involvement:

1. Can you feel swollen or enlarged regional lymph nodes? If so, do you intend to investigate them further? How?
2. Do you plan to do lymph node mapping and sentinel node sampling? If so, is this part of a clinical study?
3. Do I need to have surgery to remove a group of lymph nodes (a lymph node dissection)? If so, what are the side effects? Will there be any numbness or swelling associated with the surgery?
4. Will this be an outpatient procedure or will I need to stay overnight in the hospital?
5. Will the dissection require that a drain be inserted? For about how long?
6. When will the pathology report be available?
7. What symptoms should I call you about?
8. What should I take for pain over the next few days?

Surgery for Your Primary Melanoma   Scottish physician William Handley made recommendations in 1907 that established the style of surgical treatment of melanoma for the following fifty years.

From the autopsy findings on a single melanoma patient, he concluded that melanomas regularly penetrate the skin around them and fill the tiny lymphatic vessels. He therefore advocated making a wide local excision, about ten centimeters (or around four inches) across. The skin graft to close the surgical wound left a troublesome scar. Luckily for melanoma patients today, Handley's recommendations have been discredited by studies of many patients over the years. Narrower excisions are made now, and lymph node dissection is not performed without compelling reason.

Very wide excisions are still practiced, especially for thick melanomas, but Dr. Guerry says, "The decision for a wide excision is based on dogma, hearsay, theory, and conservatism; no one has proven that anything beyond a relatively narrow excision improves survival." Local recurrence of all but the thickest melanomas is rare after narrow excisions and is almost never the cause of disseminated disease. Death from melanoma usually occurs from microscopic disease that may have traveled even before the primary melanoma is excised to the lymph nodes and beyond, to other organs.

Before the definitive surgery is performed, diagnostic tests in addition to the physical exam, such as chest X-rays and blood work, may often be needed. An MRI or CAT scan may be done if the less technical work-up turns up something suspicious or if you are part of a study that requires it.

What Should I Look for in a Surgeon?   Both the pathology of the melanoma and the mindsets of surgeon and patient will have an important bearing on the details of your surgery. Some guidelines on the possible scope of the operation follow, but you should pick a surgeon who will pay attention to achieving satisfactory cosmetic results and who will discuss in detail what to do about lymph nodes and follow-up after surgery.

How Big Will the Surgical Wound Be?   Melanomas in the radial growth phase, whether in situ or invasive, are generally treated by

taking a band of skin and subcutaneous tissue half a centimeter to one centimeter in width. (The smallest distance
from the melanoma or the scar at the biopsy site to where
the surgeon cuts is called the margin.) Thin melanomas,
those less than a millimeter thick, can safely be treated by
taking one-centimeter margins. Melanomas that are one
to four millimeters thick are generally given one- to two-
centimeter margins. Even with a two-centimeter margin, only
a small percentage of patients will need a skin graft, which
can be troublesome cosmetically. For thick melanomas—
those exceeding four millimeters—some doctors recommend excising a margin of three centimeters or greater.

When possible, the surgeon will avoid a skin graft. Figure 25 illustrates procedures employed by Dr. David Low
(professor of surgery in the Division of Plastic Surgery at the
hospital at the University of Pennsylvania) to leave less evident scars.

What to Ask the Surgeon

1. What will my surgery be like—how big a deal will it be?
2. What margin will you aim for? You might ask your surgeon to
   draw the boundaries of the excision with a pen on your skin,
   so there won't be any surprises when you see it after surgery.
3. Will I need a skin graft? What part of my body will the graft
   come from? (Often it is from the buttocks or thighs.)
4. How incapacitated will I be afterwards? How soon can I resume normal activities?
5. Will I be an inpatient or an outpatient? If an inpatient, how
   long will I have to stay in the hospital?
6. Will I have general anesthesia? Is a local or regional anesthesia possible?
7. What about postoperative pain?

Figure 25. Surgical Techniques for Closing a Wound (David Low, M.D.)

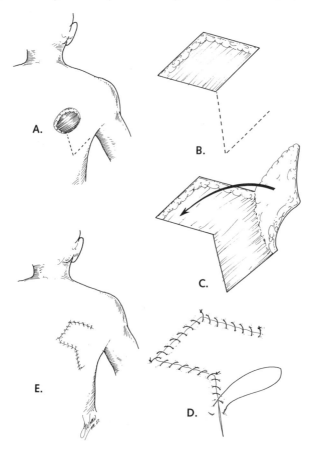

A. The patient has undergone a wide excision of a melanoma on the right upper back.
B. An adjacent skin flap is freed up and moved to close the gap.
C. The skin and underlying fat are rearranged and rotated into place.
D. The skin is stretched to fit over the excision.
E. This procedure allows for complete closure of the wound without leaving a depression in the skin and without necessitating a skin graft.

What Happens After Surgery? After you have fully re-
covered from surgery, a
schedule for follow-up examinations and diagnostic tests
will be set up for you. Follow-up guidelines will differ from
doctor to doctor and are based in part on the recognition
that the first three years after therapy are the time of highest
risk of relapse. Here is what the Pigmented Lesion Group
does for melanoma follow-up.

Melanoma patients are divided into two groups: those
with pure radial growth phase melanomas and those with
vertical growth phase melanomas or melanomas that have
metastasized to nearby skin or to regional lymph nodes. The
group with radial growth phase melanoma is checked every
six months for two years, and yearly thereafter. Because it
is highly improbable that melanoma in the radial growth
phase will metastasize, for these patients the follow-up
consists only of an exam to determine their physical status.
The doctor is on the lookout for any recurrence of melanoma at the site of the surgery or in the regional lymph node
but also for the possible development of a second primary
melanoma, which should be readily curable if it is caught
early on.

Patients with treated tumors in the vertical growth phase
or treated metastases of the lymph nodes or of skin between
the primary site and the nearest lymph nodes are seen every
three months for the first year after surgery and every four
months for the second and third years. During the fourth
through fifth years following surgery, visits are scheduled every six months; from the sixth year on, visits are annual. Patients are advised to have a chest X-ray at every other visit
for the first three years. Thereafter, X-rays are done yearly.

If during that time something new shows up, such as melanoma in a lymph node, the physician reverts to examining the patient on the original schedule.

How Do I Perform a Lymph Node Self-Exam?

You can keep an eye on your own lymph nodes, as well as on your skin, to observe any changes. Every month or so, check the lymph node nearest to where your melanoma occurred. My melanoma was on my lower leg, so I would check the crease where the thigh joins the trunk to make sure I did not have a firm lump bigger than the width of a thumbnail. If the melanoma is on your head or in the trunk area it is a little trickier to figure which lymph nodes might be involved. It is normal to feel small lymph nodes. Ask your doctor what exactly to look for when you examine your lymph nodes. Dr. Guerry cautions that because "there are no absolutes in medicine, we also let people know that even with thin melanomas they run a tiny chance of a metastasis and that we and they and their physicians ought to keep an eye (or hand) on the lymph nodes."

In 1989, I certainly didn't know whether I would be among the fortunate 95 percent who are cured or the unlucky 5 percent. The first doctor I saw told me that I had a 20 percent chance of recurrence. I am now checked only once a year for any skin changes or lymph node involvement.

(6) When Melanoma Metastasizes

> What I've got is called melanoblastoma [melanoma]
> That's a nasty thing that knows no mercy. In eight
> months, as a rule, you're done for. Just touch it with
> a knife and there'll be metastasis everywhere. It wants
> to live too, in its way, understand? I can't be cured.
> Nobody's cured. There are no cases of recovery. In
> my case, amputating my leg wouldn't be enough,
> and how can they amputate higher?—Aleksandr I.
> Solzhenitsyn, *Cancer Ward*, 1968

Vadim Zatsyrko was wrong: many are cured of melanoma, usually by surgical removal of lesions at an early stage. But melanomas in the vertical growth phase, particularly thick ones, can send spin-offs through the lymph vessels and bloodstream to other parts of the body. Although doctors can predict which melanomas are likely to spread and can make educated guesses about the timing and pattern of spread, the disease can show up in a variety of places in the body according to its own timetable.

What should be done if melanoma spreads? The answer depends on the patient, the tumor, and the treatments that are currently considered promising or effective. Because clinical researchers are constantly exploring new therapies to fight melanoma, you will want to get in touch with the sources listed here and in Appendix B to learn about the latest research and treatments. In this chapter we provide enough information to allow you and your doctor to come to a mutual decision about the best therapy for you.

What Is Metastasis?   Metastasis, the process by which cancer spreads from its starting point in the primary tumor to other parts of the body, occurs when cancer reproduces and sheds cells through the lymphatic system and blood vessels. (The word is also used to refer to a single secondary lesion or existence of the metastatic process.)

Whether and where these cells are able to grow can be explained by the *soil and seed theory,* so named, of course, because of the parallels between melanoma cells and seeds, which can take root far from the parent plant. Melanomas grow on receptive terrain. If a melanoma cell is delivered, for example, to a lymph node (potentially fertile ground), it may, after a variable period of dormancy, sprout into a colony of cancerous cells (a metastasis). This colony may in turn generate new ones.

A metastasis can thus be thought of as a collection of many cells, the descendants of the first seeds cast from the primary tumor, that form a mass at another site. Metastases sometimes manifest themselves as palpable lumps in the skin or lymph nodes, or they may occur within an internal organ and cause it to malfunction.

Two Types of Metastasis   Melanoma metastases fall into two general categories. Regional metastases, the first category, are confined to the region of the primary tumor. This region encompasses the nearby lymph nodes and the expanse of skin between the primary site and those lymph nodes. Regional metastases are thought to be established by seed-cells that travel from the primary site via tiny lymph vessels.

Distant metastases, the second category of metastatic disease, develop beyond the region of the primary melanoma. That is, they are caused by cells disseminated far from the primary site itself, the skin around it, and the regional lymph nodes. Common destinations for melanoma cells include "nonregional" skin and lymph nodes, the lungs, the liver, and the brain. Melanoma cells spread after first entering either small blood vessels at the primary site or in the regional lymph nodes.

Treatments for Regional Metastases   Metastases confined to skin in the region of the primary site are usually surgically removed. Equivalent techniques are sometimes used, including laser surgery (to vaporize certain surface metastases) and the injection of inflammatory agents.

In the case of multiple metastases in the skin and subcutaneous tissue of an extremity, the whole limb may be treated through *regional perfusion*. During this procedure, a tourniquet is applied to isolate the blood supply of the limb from the rest of your body's circulation. The diseased arm or leg is then infused with heated cancer-killing drugs. The drugs are injected into the artery supplying the limb and are then removed through the vein. Regional perfusion, by treating only the affected limb, avoids the systemic toxicity of chemotherapy. Unfortunately, it will not take care of melanoma cells that have migrated elsewhere in the body. The procedure, which must be performed by a specially trained surgical oncologist, requires general anesthesia and several days of hospitalization. (See Chapter 5 for a more detailed discussion on treatment of melanoma that has spread to regional lymph nodes.)

Adjuvant therapy is any treatment intended to supplement the surgical removal of cancer. Generally, it is given in a way that affects the whole body: it is designed to kill disease that may have escaped to other parts of the body even before the primary tumor or diseased lymph nodes could be removed. Doctors call on adjuvant therapy when the disease is statistically likely to have metastasized but no evidence of distant disease is actually uncovered when the patient is scanned from head to toe.

When the risk of discovering subsequent metastasis is high, two precautionary steps can be taken. First, the surgeon removes the primary lesion and sometimes the regional lymph nodes. Next, a doctor, usually a medical oncologist, administers an adjuvant agent with the aim of killing any melanoma cells remaining elsewhere—and, ideally, preventing the disease from ever returning. Applying adjuvant therapy is like putting weed killer on a garden.

Just as with breast cancer, where lumpectomy and radiation are followed by chemotherapy and hormonal therapy to increase the probability of a complete cure, some melanomas are treated through surgery followed by adjuvant therapy. But unlike with breast cancer, it has been difficult with melanoma to find a treatment that will kill undetectable metastases.

Figuring out who will benefit from adjuvant therapy has been relatively straightforward: people whose melanomas are thicker than four millimeters or whose regional lymph nodes (or especially several nodes) are involved are the potential beneficiaries. The problem has been finding something that works.

Alpha-Interferon

Alpha-interferon is a biotechnically synthesized protein that is identical to a protein the body produces when it fights off viral infections. Alpha-interferon is the only agent currently approved by the Federal Drug Administration as adjuvant therapy for melanoma patients. The approval was based on a clinical research study, published in the January 1996 *Journal of Clinical Oncology,* in which patients with thick melanomas or regional lymph node involvement received either high doses of alpha-interferon or no adjuvant therapy. Five years later, 46 percent of the patients treated with interferon were still alive, as opposed to only 37 percent of the untreated patients.[1]

When given in the high doses that are apparently necessary to treat melanoma effectively, alpha-interferon has many side effects. Patients taking it feel at first as though they have the flu. This effect wears off with time and can be alleviated with other medicines. Alpha-interferon may cause severe toxic damage to the liver, significant decreases in blood count, hair loss, and neuropsychological reactions.

A one-year course of alpha-interferon (the recommended duration) costs between $15,000 and $30,000 for the medicine alone. Other medical costs can add to this. The first twenty doses are given intravenously in a doctor's office five days out of seven for a month. Blood tests need to be done frequently. Medical insurance should pay for alpha-interferon as well as the other expenses incurred.

You will need to discuss with your doctor, probably a medical or surgical oncologist, whether alpha-interferon is for you. If you are twenty-eight years old and have a 10 percent chance of a cure you may be willing to put up with the side-effects and the expense of this treatment. If you are seventy-four and have a 70 percent chance of survival, you probably aren't going to want to endure a year of feeling miserable. This is a very individual decision, best made by you and your doctor. Keep in mind that the older and more infirm you are, the less favorable your risk-to-benefit ratio.

Are Other Adjuvant Therapies Available?
Quite a number of adjuvant therapies are undergoing preliminary exploration or clinical trial. Many are less toxic than alpha-interferon, although none has yet been rigorously proved to be even as modestly effective as the synthetic protein. One kind of adjuvant therapy is a vaccine derived from your metastasis itself. Usually the tumor has to be at least two and a half centimeters (about an inch) in diameter to reproduce enough melanoma cells for a vaccine. Other vaccines are made from other people's melanoma cells that are grown then killed or from synthetic molecules identical to certain structures on melanoma cells.

Be sure to check the Internet (Oncolink, for example) for other adjuvant programs as they become available, or call the National Cancer Institute Hotline at 800-4-CANCER. The hotline provides up-to-date information on clinical trials for your stage of disease and programs in your geographical area. If transportation is a problem, the American Cancer Society may be able to help out locally. Transportation by corporate jet is even available at no charge for certain cancer patients who need to travel some distance for treatment. (See Appendix B.)

Treatments for Disseminated Melanoma

Melanoma that appears throughout the skin or has spread to the internal organs is, in the vast majority of cases, incurable. The goal in treating most patients who have reached this stage is to blunt the symptoms of the disease (through palliative treatment) and, when possible, to prolong survival with reasonable quality of life. The therapeutic plan for an individual patient will depend on prior treatment; the location and extent of the metastatic disease; the patient's age, general health, and personal wishes; and the availability of clinical research studies on new kinds of therapy. The following story concerns one of Dr. Guerry's patients who had widely disseminated melanoma.

Lisa had a suspicious-looking mole removed from the skin over her cheekbone in 1989. The pathology report identified it as melanoma. Re-excision of the area around the melanoma was advised by her doctor, and she had that second surgery performed.

Lisa first came to see Dr. Guerry after she discovered a swollen lymph node in her neck, about four years after the primary melanoma had been excised. The surgeon removed a lymph node, which turned out to be positive for melanoma. She then had the adjacent lymph nodes removed; the procedure confirmed that only one lymph node was involved.

A year later while Lisa was at a soccer game watching her son play, she discovered that bumps had popped up all over her head. Then a lump appeared on her back.

She returned to see Dr. Guerry. After diagnostic tests she was found to have widespread melanoma: her skin, her lungs, her kidneys, and the coverings of her brain had become involved. She decided on chemotherapy, after thoroughly discussing the toxicity and effectiveness of the treatment with Dr. Guerry. After two rounds of chemotherapy in the hospital, she appeared to be free of disease. She nevertheless completed the entire chemotherapy course of six monthly treatments. Then, two months later, metastases developed within her brain, and she underwent surgery and radiation to it. She is now feeling fine and has been free of disease for more than a year. Dr. Guerry helped Lisa get into an experimental vaccine program in California, to which she travels monthly.

Chemotherapy and Biological Therapies   Although chemotherapy sometimes produces dramatic regression of disseminated melanoma like Lisa's, it only rarely results in long-term survival. Indeed, in a recent review of chemotherapy for cancer

in advanced stages, melanoma patients were classed with those who could expect only "minor response—no demonstrable prolongation of survival" from chemotherapy.[2]

New therapies that stimulate the immune system to attack melanoma or that choke off the specialized blood vessels supplying metastases may offer effective therapy in the future. Such biological therapies—for example, vaccines and immunological hormones called cytokines—offer hope for melanoma treatment. It now seems that in a few patients, disease may actually melt away, after it has been treated with interleukin-2. This kind of remission has been sustained over years in some patients. At a recent oncology conference, Dr. Stephen Rosenberg of the National Cancer Institute documented some remissions associated with a melanoma vaccine trial he heads. At a series of lectures ("New Developments in Cancer Therapy: Focus on Surgical Oncology") at the University of Pennsylvania Cancer Center, he showed "before and after" slides of patients, first with melanoma metastases protruding from their bodies, then after treatment with a synthetic vaccine, when the tumors had disappeared.[3] He expressed merely guarded optimism, however: as with interleukin-2 therapy, the tumors shrank in only a very small percentage of the patients he treated.

Clinical Trials   There is no standard therapy for suspected or evident disseminated disease. To learn about current clinical trials, patients should get in touch with the National Cancer Institute. In 1997 seventeen trials of adjuvant therapy were under way for people with Stage III melanoma (that is, with disease apparently confined to the regional lymph nodes) and fifty-five trials for Stage IV patients (with documented disseminated disease)—an indication of the widespread interest in finding new therapies for melanoma.

To qualify for any given trial, you must meet certain requirements. Most trials require you to be eighteen years or older. In general, you can't be too sick when you enter the trial. And patients with metastases in certain locations—the brain, for instance—may be disqualified. Other research protocols require that you not have had such previous treatment as chemotherapy or vaccines, or that a certain amount of time must have elapsed since your last treatment. The National Cancer Institute's PDQ database (800-4-CANCER) has a listing of all of the trials and entry criteria. Call to request their pamphlet *What Are Clinical Trials All About?*

Questions to Ask Before Joining a Clinical Trial

1. What is the purpose of this study? Who is sponsoring it? How is it reviewed for safety?
2. What kinds of tests and treatments must I go through? What are the potential side-effects? Get specific details about how the drug is administered and what any relevant studies to date have shown about side-effects.
3. Will some participants receive a placebo and others get the real thing? Many studies are set up to determine how patients who receive the treatment do by comparison with those who receive nothing. Also, many trials are "double-blind": neither the doctor nor the patient knows what the patient is getting.

You can leave the trial at any time. Also, if it is clear that you are getting worse, the trial will end for you.

What About Alternative Medicine?   Because there seem
to be very few effec-
tive treatments of melanoma, you may find yourself looking
at alternative medicine. Many alternative treatments are un-
proven, so be careful about deciding to try one. Always discuss any alternative treatment and its possible benefits with
your doctor—especially because it may conflict with your
current traditional therapy.

7   Tending to Your Spirits

Can I find inside each day a little oasis of joy? Even with the fear, can I attach myself to the moment? For inspiration I look to family, friends, and new celebrations.
—Carolyn Marks

Psychologically, the waiting is the hardest part for a person dealing with melanoma—or any other cancer. Over and over, normal life is put on hold because of the disease. First, the patient is in limbo until the initial biopsy results are made available. Then comes the nervous waiting from check-up to check-up to learn whether any recurrence has been detected. If the disease does make a comeback, the patient must wait again, this time for the results of the diagnostic tests.

Meanwhile, the mind works overtime, as the patient imagines every conceivable outcome, from best to worst. To make matters still more difficult, family members and health care providers may overreact during this process or may be unable to decide on the most desirable course of treatment. All these factors contribute to the patient's feeling out of control and helpless to deal with the situation. In the past, cancer patients were often passive observers of their care who were out of the loop. The physician and family members kept the details of the patient's treatment and life expectancy a closely guarded secret. Fortunately, the trend these days is for patients to be actively involved in their treatment. I highly recommend that you make a point of working in full partnership with your physician. Not only will you receive better care, but you will take a step toward conquering your fear of the unknown by gathering knowledge and gain some measure of control during a very vulnerable time in your life.

In coping with melanoma, you will probably manage your fear in whatever style you generally adopt in a crisis. You should proceed in the way that makes you feel most comfortable. The resources and ideas I present in this chapter are intended to make you feel more at ease in dealing with your melanoma, no matter what your prognosis.

Finding the Right Doctor　The first step toward taking care of your melanoma is choosing a doctor you feel confidence in. At the second of the two university teaching hospitals I visited I found the right melanoma specialist. A few years later, when I moved to the West Coast, I had to locate a new doctor for my follow-up visits. Luckily, I found a great family doctor. Because she coincidentally had a close relative with melanoma, she was acutely aware of the importance of my check-ups and knew what to look for.

You might be fortunate enough to find a dermatologist or family physician in your community who is knowledgeable about melanoma. It is worth the trouble to travel a certain

distance if you need to, though, to find the right doctor.
Even if you have a low-risk melanoma, as I had, and certainly if you are at high risk for recurrence, you should seek
out a specialist who is well versed in the field. At the same
time, make sure that both the specified pathological characteristics of the melanoma and the diagnosis are correct.
You don't want to risk getting inappropriate or inadequate
treatment.

A physician who deals with melanoma on a regular basis
will probably be better informed about treatments and
more relaxed in talking to you about the disease. Melanoma
specialists are frequently able to link up with a qualified
network of surgeons, pathologists, oncologists, and mental
health professionals and thus provide you with more comprehensive care. It might be a good idea to go for your initial
evaluation and surgery at a specialized clinic and then have
your follow-up check-ups locally.

Needless to say, your doctor's professional expertise will
be critical. The practitioner's personality may also matter to
you, although it does not necessarily give an indication of
medical proficiency. You will probably be able to gauge the
doctor's willingness to give you a say in your own treatment,
to treat you like a respected colleague as you work together.

Where do you find a doctor who will cooperate with you
in this way? A teaching hospital will usually have a good
melanoma team. A hospital that has been designated a Comprehensive Cancer Center by the National Cancer Institute
offers additional advantages, because it has demonstrated
that it has a strong research program that supports its clinical practice. In looking for a doctor, call ahead and talk with
the nursing staff. You can often get a feel from the initial

contact for how the clinic or practice operates. Nurses are also an excellent resource—they may be able to recommend a good doctor.

Finding Peace of Mind　If you're lucky, the physician or melanoma clinic you visit may include care for your mind as well as for your body. The Melanoma Center at the University of California at San Francisco provides psychological counseling and evaluation for all patients. Before coming in for the initial appointment, patients are notified in a letter that their first visit will include a meeting with a psychologist. They are reassured that it's routine and that they're not being singled out.

Clinical psychologist Andrew Kneier sees all new patients who come to both the Melanoma Center and the Breast Care Center. Most have just been diagnosed with cancer, but some are coming in because they have experienced a recurrence.

Dr. Kneier says, "They're scared and have just learned of their diagnosis. I try to pay attention to the emotional impact of this and how they're coping and adjusting to it, by providing education, support, and guidance. Patients can express their worry and get some perspective on it. I've been doing this for fourteen years and have become a conduit for information—I share with new patients what I've learned from a large group of people who have passed this way before them."

Dr. Kneier also runs two monthly melanoma support groups that bring together high- and low-risk patients. According to Kneier, "The nature of the groups is really peer support and learning positive ways to cope and provide an outlet to express fears. Deaths do occur in the group. It's a moving experience. It smacks them in the face that this could happen to them, but they don't want to be shielded from that; they want to confront those fears."

If your clinic or doctor doesn't bring up psychological care as a part of treatment and you feel the need, request a recommendation for a therapist who counsels cancer patients. At the Pigmented Lesion Clinic, patients are asked during the initial screening process whether they are feeling distressed about their illness. As Dr. Guerry remarks, "Good physicians can usually sense distress in patients and figure out which ones need their spirits attended to. I often say to patients, 'How is your head doing?' Issues of the psyche come up. It only takes a question or two to figure out if the patient has issues to deal with."

If the patient wants to discuss unresolved issues with a therapist or if during the examination the physician detects a need for counseling, the patient will be referred to a specialist.

Dr. Arlene Houldin, a psychosocial oncology consultant at the University of Pennsylvania's Cancer Center, sees patients who have metastases or recurrent disease. "Often," she explains, they "feel they are living with a time bomb, which may send them into counseling." She frequently sees the patient and then the other family members as a group before seeing all of them together, because she recognizes that individuals may want to raise certain issues without their relatives present.

Dr. Houldin says, "I support people through a tough time—basically by providing supportive therapy, teaching

coping techniques, decision making, and problem-solving
skills—and assist in resolving family issues. There's frequently a sublevel of anger and blame that needs to be dealt
with, sometimes involving blame for sun-worshiping habits
much like the guilt associated with smoking and lung cancer. Melanoma is horribly disruptive, because it often hits
younger people who are just raising their families, heavily
into career goals, with lots of financial burdens; and sometimes they are even caring for older family members, and
suddenly they're struck down by this illness, disrupting
their own personal plans and the family in a major way. So
melanoma can involve a lot more family issues to deal with
than some other cancers."

Coping Styles   Dr. Guerry has found from working with
patients facing life-threatening illness that
"you can't try to suddenly change a person's lifetime coping
mechanism; professionals working with cancer patients
shouldn't try to take their usual way of coping and break it
down and change it—they need to be aware and respectful
of that."

Dr. Houldin agrees that "this is not the time to confront
patients with ways to cope that are foreign to them, because
if you do, you will lose their trust." She adds, "You try to
process the fears and provide support even for the person
whose style is to avoid rather than confront the emotional
issues."

Dr. Guerry points out that there isn't "one coping style
or another that changes the biology of the disease, but a
coping style where you stick your head in the ground and

you don't get good medical follow-up may cause you to miss the opportunity of finding something you can do that will help you—like taking out a regional lymph node that has melanoma in it, or joining a clinical trial. With denial of the disease, you may miss the opportunity for emotional stability or spiritual growth that comes from working through whatever happens with loved ones, friends, and counselors and physicians. To miss this is to miss something important."

Places You Can Go for Help Sometimes if you can get away from it all, you can gain some perspective on your situation. You may want to enroll in a residential program where you can get intensive help in coping with all aspects of your illness. Many programs provide group therapy, nutritional counseling, massage, yoga, relaxation techniques, and suggestions about adjusting to chemotherapy and other treatments, all in a supportive environment. Some places offering beautiful vistas and comfortable lodgings with all the amenities can cost upwards of $1,500 a week, but occasionally they have a few scholarships available.

Others are more reasonably priced and may offer the opportunity to refocus yourself, take your mind off your illness, and develop your self-esteem and potential for growth during this time of crisis. Outward Bound, although primarily known for wilderness survival training and rock climbing courses, will tailor programs for a particular group— say, a melanoma support group. (See Appendix B.) Not all the offerings are rugged outdoor experiences: some indoor programs are featured. The usual cost is about $125 a day, including food and lodging for the travel program. Outward Bound does not provide programs for individuals; you must sign up as part of a group.

Other, similar intensive programs exist (again, see Appendix B); some are covered by health insurance and some aren't. You can sometimes persuade your insurance company to provide coverage, on the grounds that the program will help you get through a difficult time in better form and possibly forestall future therapy expenses.

If you'd rather stick close to home and have someplace comforting to visit if you feel the need, bear in mind the Wellness Community. Its stated mission is "helping people with cancer fight for their recovery by providing psychological and emotional support as an adjunct to conventional medical treatment, at no charge." It offers drop-in and regularly scheduled support groups, networking groups for people with specific types of cancer, lectures by experts in oncology, relaxation and visualization exercises, social gatherings, and, most important, "laughter, joy and hope," as the brochure puts it.

I visited the Philadelphia chapter of the Wellness Community and immediately felt at home when the resident dog therapist, Max, greeted me at the door. Program director Laurie Curtis explained that Max, a stray she adopted, provides unconditional love to visitors and staff and helps maintain the home-away-from-home atmosphere.

The Wellness Community group therapy sessions, she told me, "help the patient stay actively involved and avoid the assumption that the therapist is the expert." The groups steer people away from discussing the specifics of their treatments and instead work on how patients are feeling about their illness. The daily calendar is full of activities, including t'ai chi, yoga, meditation, and cancer-related seminars. Special events are scheduled, too, such as a picnic in the park or a laugh fest. The Wellness Community offers support groups for different lifestyles and situations—for single people, couples, women only, men only, family members, newcomers, and long-term survivors. All the programs are free of charge. The headquarters will help you find a chapter near you. (See Appendix B.)

The American Cancer Society (ACS, telephone 800-ACS-2345) offers a wide range of educational materials and listings of support groups in your locality. The ACS can also provide equipment for home care and other support services.

Another good source of information is the hospital where you had surgery or treatment. Nurses are frequently ready to help you deal with the psychological aspects of melanoma or to assist you in finding someone within the hospital community who can provide counseling. Hospital social workers, too, often have a wealth of information at their fingertips about local resources and home care.

There's Strength in Numbers   Not all people are cut out for support groups. Many of us find it hard to open up to a group of people we hardly know. I found joining a support group a daunting undertaking after my initial diagnosis of melanoma, partly because I was afraid someone in the group would die.

That being said, support groups do often provide a safe environment where, as one participant put it, "you can't scare each other." A good many of the group members may already have weathered what you are going through. They will usually allow you to express whatever you want to without reacting judgmentally, something friends and family may have trouble doing.

Some studies strongly suggest that people who participate in support groups live longer than those who don't. One of the most compelling is a recent study by psychiatrist David Spiegel at Stanford University. In trying to *disprove* that psychological factors affected cancer, he looked at vital statistics comparing participants in his breast cancer support groups with nonparticipants. He found that the women in the support group survived eighteen months longer on average than those who didn't join a support group.

Spiegel attributes the increased longevity primarily to what he calls the "grandmother effect." A similar mechanism is thought to explain why married men live longer than single men: people who feel that others care about them and who are being taken care of often avoid harmful habits and eat, sleep, and exercise well, thus fortifying the body's ability to fight illness.[1] In a new study Spiegel is monitoring the immune function, in an attempt to confirm the results of the first study and possibly find other reasons for the greater longevity of support group participants.

In another study Fawzy I. Fawzy, a psychiatrist at the University of California at Los Angeles, examined the outcome of sixty-eight melanoma cases and found that patients who were not in support groups had a higher death rate than those who were receiving psychological support from a group.[2]

If you decide to join a support group, you may have trouble finding one specifically geared to melanoma patients. Just this year, I helped initiate a melanoma support group at the Philadelphia chapter of the Wellness Community. You may want to start a group yourself. It should meet at least once a month. The biggest expense will be the group facilitator's fee, but don't stint on that: smooth group functioning may depend on the guidance of someone with a solid counseling background. Each participant could chip in a nominal amount to cover the expense. You may be able to hold meetings in a hospital waiting room or a library at no charge. Doctors or clinics that treat melanoma may provide names of potential members.

Your Family How your family reacts to your diagnosis may present unexpected problems. Families under stress communicate inefficiently or in bizarre ways. You may find loved ones responding with unaccustomed behavior—for example, denial and avoidance. (The same goes for friends.) However your family ordinarily functions, honest, open communication is ultimately the most comforting. All of us have a sixth sense about when people aren't being candid with us, and especially when those closest to us are being insincere. Dr. Guerry finds that "one of the things families make the mistake of doing is hiding information. So in the communication dodging, either the patient or family member thinks things are worse than they are, and then the whole family avoids talking about the issues. My single piece of advice would be to talk to each other and be up front when you do."

It is often hardest to communicate with family members, because of long-established patterns of interaction. Sometimes emotional ties may even be too strong. According to Dr. Kneier, "Patients don't feel as comfortable talking to their friends and family about their fears, because they're always getting pep talks. 'Keep a positive attitude,' they're urged. It's well intended by family but misguided, because it doesn't validate their [the patients'] feelings, and then they feel depressed because they're not supposed to worry, and then they get concerned that a recurrence may result from these feelings, and it is a big trap to get caught in." If you are having problems talking about your illness with your family, a therapist who specializes in crisis counseling can facilitate better communication between you and them.

The Mind-Body Connection Another psychological trap, akin to the family cheerleading already mentioned, originates with the mistaken belief that a person can get cancer (or provoke a recurrence) by not coping right or by handling stress badly. The cancer-prone personality is a myth. You cannot get cancer—or aggravate cancer once you have it—by thinking particular thoughts.

Dr. Kneier explains, "All this talk of mind over body makes patients feel guilty and responsible for their cancer: maybe they caused it by not coping with life the right way.

Our society makes them feel that their survival is up to them. But there really isn't any proof of this."

Dr. Houldin points out that many patients, influenced by publications that stress positive thinking, are filled with guilt because they imagine that the inability to cope has brought on their cancer. "While those books can be enormously helpful, sometimes they carry a hidden message of guilt: 'If I'm not positive all the time, my cancer will get worse or come back.' Clearly, the scientific evidence doesn't show that. People should not be beating themselves up at this time of crisis. Unfortunately, some families will use this mind-body theory to keep patients under control, saying, 'You're not being positive enough' (or, 'you're not being cheerful enough'), 'so you won't get better.' Here people are, dealing with the diagnosis of the illness, the treatment and the uncertainty of having it, and then they have to be positive all of the time. Cancer patients need to be given permission to be upset and grieve and vent their negative feelings."

Worrying About Your Body   While you're allowing yourself to be upset, give yourself permission to be a hypochondriac, too. As if it isn't enough that you are dealing with all this pressure to be happy and positive, you are also forced to tune in to your body more than ever before. Your confidence in your immune system is shaky; after all, if your body let you down once, it might do it again. Every little symptom you develop may drive you crazy thinking that this is a recurrence or spread of melanoma. Doctors inexperienced in cancer treatment may not be sensitive to this issue and may either dismiss your concerns or scare you needlessly. I remember initially thinking that swollen lymph nodes in my neck might be metastasized melanoma. Luckily, the nurses at the Pigmented Lesion Clinic were quite used to reassuring patients about similar concerns and calmed me down.

Another time, my general practitioner said my tonsils were inflamed and that because they were a type of lymph node, the inflammation might be connected with a recurrence of the melanoma. In a panic, I called Dr. Guerry, only to be reassured that my symptoms were "astoundingly unlikely" to indicate a recurrence. Still, if you have a gut feeling that something *is* going on, don't worry about looking ridiculous. Talk about it with your doctor and get it checked, so you can stop worrying. And switch doctors if your queries are met with patronizing remarks or dismissed too easily. Sooner or later your feelings about your body will normalize.

In the Long Run   You should also bear in mind that your doctor is a human being who doesn't have any magical powers to cure you and certainly doesn't have all the answers all of the time. Giving yourself permission to be upset will actually help regulate your emotional reactions. It's okay to feel sorry for yourself and to feel scared. It will be especially beneficial if you can confront the issues that upset and frighten you and then process them emotionally. Don't be afraid to ask for help from either a professional therapist or those close to you. This is a lot to handle on your own.

Many cancer patients are ultimately thankful to be brought face to face with their own mortality, because for the first time in their lives they get their priorities straight. The other challenges encountered in life may seem trivial by comparison. And despite the initial quaking you feel, you will emerge from this ordeal on a stronger foundation than you ever imagined.

8

Future Promise: Prevention of Melanoma

Hee is a better physician that keeps diseases off us than hee that cures them being on us. Prevention is so much better than healing, because it saves us the labor of being sick.—Thomas Adams, 17th century

In the long run, medical science should aim to prevent disease rather than merely try to cure people who already suffer from it. But melanoma can be prevented only if people are made aware of its causes and if they will change their behavior to avoid getting it. Unfortunately, many people are skeptical or unaware that sunshine is a potential carcinogen. Basking in the sun seems an enticing way to relax, and tanned skin is considered appealing. Hence, our recreational lifestyles still revolve around the sunniest places and parts of the day. It's worth exploring how we might change these attitudes and work to prevent melanoma.

Clueless in the U.S.A. In the United States large segments of the population don't have a clue about what melanoma is or what causes it—so they naturally lack the motivation to try to prevent it. Public education about prevention and detection remains a formidable task.

The results of a survey released in May 1996 by the U.S. Centers for Disease Control and Prevention and the American Academy of Dermatology noted that a whopping 74 percent of Americans between the ages of eighteen and twenty-four did not know what melanoma was; among those aged twenty-five to forty-four, 42 percent had no knowledge about it; 30 percent of people between forty-five and sixty-four and 31 percent of those sixty-five and over were ignorant about the disease.[1] The showing in the United Kingdom was still worse: only 26 percent of the adult population knew anything about melanoma. It is interesting to compare these figures with those for Victoria, Australia, where 91 percent of the residents surveyed knew about melanoma.[2]

Australians know they have to deal a blow to the staggeringly high incidence of melanoma in their country. As a consequence, Australia has become an innovative leader in educational and preventive programs. The Anti-Cancer Council of Victoria recently developed SunSmart, a sharply focused campaign for the prevention and early detection of melanoma. The program literature and ads feature a seagull named Sid, who urges all Australians to "slip on a shirt, slop on some sunscreen, and slap on a hat." The efforts are paying off with a measurable increase in awareness and with behavioral changes.[3]

What Steps Are We Taking?

The Centers for Disease Control and Prevention in

Atlanta awarded $1.2 million to the American Academy of
Dermatology (AAD) for the years 1995 to 1997, to follow Australia's lead in providing a comprehensive educational program to spread the message: "Sun protection may save your
life." So far the AAD has come up with several programs to
prevent melanoma. (See Figure 26.) A relatively new program, Melanoma Monday, is a media blitz that is held by
the AAD on the first Monday in May in New York City, to
raise awareness about melanoma and encourage Americans
to begin a lifelong habit of regular skin self-examinations.
Melanoma Monday also marks the beginning of Melanoma /
Skin Cancer Detection and Prevention Month. During this
designated month and throughout the year, more than two
thousand volunteer dermatologists offer free screenings in
hospitals, at private offices, and at health fairs. In addition,
as part of the effort to educate Americans about melanoma
and sun exposure, billboards, radio spots, and television
commercials are starting to hit the airwaves.

Children: It's Never Too Early to Begin Their Education

How early can we start educating children about melanoma? Actually, we should
start by educating parents before children are born. During
the traditional prenatal or postnatal education classes, parents can be taught about protecting their children from
the sun.

Very early on, parents can set an example for their children by taking appropriate precautions against overexposure to the sun. It is important for parents to realize that an

Figure 26. American Academy of Dermatology Advertisements

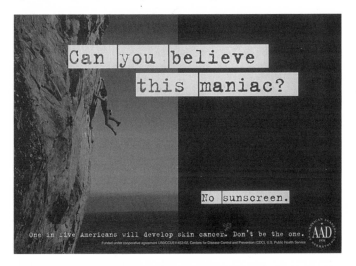

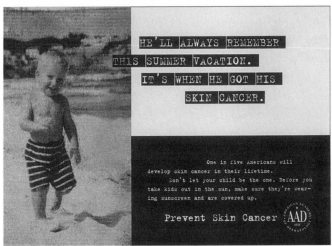

attitude of "do as I say, not as I do" confuses the message for children.

If avoiding excessive sun becomes an acceptable goal in our culture, the behaviors associated with it will become the norm. As my pediatrician, Tom Fitzpatrick, says, "Putting sunscreen lotion on should be just as automatic as putting seatbelts on children." Tom always incorporates a skin exam into my children's annual physical. He checks their skin for sun damage and makes suggestions about sunscreen and avoidance of sun. The AAD has formed an alliance with the American Academy of Pediatrics to further this type of education for children and their caretakers. Education specialists assert that behavior taught early in life is the least resistant to change.

Educational efforts in a preschool setting have proved effective for children as young as four years old. A program created for preschoolers by the Arizona Cancer Center called Be Sun-Safe has been measured for effectiveness in a randomized trial. The term *skin cancer* was avoided in the program because it was considered too frightening for four-year-olds, but the importance of sun safety and taking care of your body was emphasized.[4]

After taking part in puppet shows, hat-making activities, and shade-finding games (often led by teenage or senior volunteers), the children showed definite changes in attitude about the sun. The Be Sun-Safe program message was reinforced by observance of recommended precautions (like putting on sunscreen lotion and hats) when the children went outside to play. Children were aware that recess was scheduled for a time when the sun was low in the sky.[5]

When School Lets Out   Summer camps are of special concern to Dr. Howard Koh, director of cancer prevention at Boston University: "Camps are where every summer millions of American kids just get fried." At camp, children may be overexposed to sun during *all* the prime-time hours (that is, between ten in the morning and three in the afternoon), whereas in school they are exposed for an hour or less at a time. Public health programs have been initiated in Massachusetts and Hawaii to try to change summer camp habits; they reward campers for using sun protection and avoiding prime-time sun.

A sun safety policy needs to be embedded in the curriculum for all organized activities for children, whether the sports programs of the YMCA and others or those of public school systems. Most of these organizations have drawn up rules of behavior based on safety considerations, and it would seem logical to include sun safety recommendations among them. Teachers can hardly go around applying sunscreen lotion to students (that would attract lawsuits), but getting children to wear a hat outdoors on sunny days—a requirement in Australian schools—may be a simpler way to promote sun protection.

Children can't seek shade if there isn't any. Playgrounds need to be redesigned with this limitation in mind. Shading with trees, trellises, or awnings would provide some respite, and some improvement over the black-top playground wide open to the sun. At most grade schools outdoor recess is at high noon, the worst possible time of day as far as sun exposure is concerned. Recess could easily be scheduled for early morning or late afternoon to minimize midday exposure.

It is imperative that daycare settings, like schools, put sun-avoidance strategies into effect. I know of one large hospital-based daycare and kindergarten where parents are asked to apply sunscreen to their children before dropping them off in the morning. In addition, parents may provide sunscreen lotion to be applied by teachers later in the day. According to the director, there are no national guidelines or suggestions on sun protection for daycare administrators to follow.

In addition to protecting your children from sun exposure, it is a good idea to examine their skin. Keep track of moles, and have their physician check any skin changes you are worried about. Teach your children as they get older how to examine their own skin, as well.

Weaning Teens from the Sun The American Academy of Dermatology survey found that 74 percent of seventeen-to-twenty-five-year-olds had no knowledge of what melanoma is. They are also very much at risk for developing nonmelanoma skin cancer. People in this age group are the least likely to protect themselves from the sun and the most likely to suffer from overexposure to it.[6] Since most young adults believe they are immortal, a warning about the dangers of sunbathing tends to produce the "who cares" response. It might work better to appeal to their vanity by pointing out that if they get too much sun, their skin is going to be permanently wrinkled and they will look old before their time.[7]

A priority of the SunSmart program in Australia is to help young adults change attitudes about sun behavior. The program managers recognize that "among young adults, issues such as appearance, fashion, acceptability, image and behavior are a minefield through which we must tread with great care, for to put a foot wrong could be very counterproductive."[8]

What About Men?   Dr. Ken Goldberg, founder of the Men's Health Network, noting that men's lives are seven years shorter on average than women's, points out that men seldom take care of their bodies the way they take care of their cars or their computers. As we mentioned in Chapter 4, men seldom find melanomas. It is usually the women in their lives who do so and who get them to the doctor.

The mortality rate from melanoma is higher for men than it is for women, although the rate of occurrence is about the same for both sexes. In fact, men over fifty have the highest melanoma fatality rates. Many men delay in seeking a doctor's advice and are likely to ignore—or not even notice—a change in their skin until it is too late.

A New Attitude   A profound cultural shift in attitudes about the sun needs to take place. Our society is still bent on sun worshiping. Dermatologists stress that there is no such thing as a "healthy tan," yet a survey mentioned in a pamphlet put out by the AAD shows that two-thirds of U.S. residents think people look better with a tan and more than half say they "work on a tan" when they go outdoors.[9] A dermatologist I interviewed remarked that it remains macho for men to take off their shirts in the sun and that women often avoid using sunscreen products because they want to "have color."

Attitudes are changing, but only extremely gradually. As Dr. Koh points out, "If sun attitudes can be compared to smoking, remember: the surgeon general's report about the hazards of smoking came out in 1964, and a quarter of our citizens still smoke cigarettes, so it may take a very long time for change to occur."[10]

At one time, Australia had cultural values similar to ours about sun, but in 1980 it became very serious about educating its citizens to think differently, in an attempt to slow its melanoma rate, the highest in the world at more than thirty cases per hundred thousand people.

To induce those who are hooked on sunbathing to change, it may be necessary to look (as Australia did) to certain groups that wield great influence—starting with the media and the sports industry. If those powerful organizations were to reinforce some simple changes in lifestyle, a lot of fans would heed the message.

Concerned Australians have succeeded in getting the co-operation of organized sports to reschedule activities such as their much-loved cricket matches away from the scorching noon hour. Such techniques could work well in the United States. We should start with Little League baseball, and then extend our efforts to professional football, baseball, tennis, and other multimillion-dollar sports.

The media and the advertising industry can exercise powerful public persuasion. It's a good sign that the Coppertone ads, which formerly depicted a dog pulling down a bikini bottom to expose a child's tan line, now show the dog pulling at the child's oversized shirt to protect her from sun. Also, magazines are starting to feature untanned models much more frequently than in previous decades. The American Academy of Dermatology has its own ads up and running nationally. One television spot shows a woman, an obvious sun worshiper, toweling off from an ocean swim to the tune of "I've Got You Under My Skin." As she dries her shoulder, viewers can see that she has a sizable melanoma. The voice-over, meanwhile, discusses early melanoma detection. Another ad shows a shirtless red-haired boy riding his tricycle down a major highway. As the trucks whiz by, the announcer comments that the child is more likely to be struck down by skin cancer than by a car or truck.

A Different Sun   Chlorofluorocarbons released into the atmosphere over the last few decades, primarily from manufacturing chemicals and air-conditioning and refrigeration equipment, have eaten away at the ozone layer that protects us from the UV-B in solar radiation. The hole in the ozone is about the size of Europe.

We must be more careful about our own and our children's sun exposure than we were a decade ago. Scientists warn that the Earth is now entering the decade in which the planet will be exposed to the greatest dose of ultraviolet radiation from the sun.

According to Daniel Albritton, director of the National Oceanic and Atmospheric Administration's Aeronomy Lab, "We'll feel the greatest impact of ozone depletion over the next 10 years and then, as the ozone layer repairs itself from decreased use of chlorofluorocarbons and other industrial chemicals, the situation will begin to improve."[11]

The Argument for Tanning
Some say that tanning protects your skin from melanoma, and Dr. Guerry concurs that gradual, natural tanning probably acts as a weak sunblock and may provide some protection from melanoma. But you won't find him or other doctors recommending that you work on a tan. Sun exposure damages your skin, whether your tan is acquired naturally or from a tanning salon.

Excessive exposure to ultraviolet (UV) radiation from either source not only makes your skin ugly in the long run by creasing it and drying it out until it looks like leather but also without a doubt constitutes a risk factor for melanoma and other skin cancers. Exposure also has a systemic effect on your body; for example, it causes some suppression of the immune system.

Distinguishing Between the Rays
Only 6 percent of the solar radiation that reaches the Earth is ultraviolet light. UV light is invisible but powerful enough to damage skin permanently. Two known types of ultraviolet light that penetrate the Earth's atmosphere cause sunburn: UV-A and UV-B. The latest studies have found that both kinds of rays are implicated in causing the damage that leads to nonmelanoma skin cancer and melanoma.

UV-A is also considered the major cause of skin aging: it

damages collagen, elastin, and other structural molecules. UV-B is thought to be the primary cause of melanoma. Sunscreens have always protected against UV-B, and recently they have been formulated to screen out UV-A rays, as well.

Do Sunscreens Really Protect You from Melanoma?

Prevention specialists feel that sunscreen should be used only as an adjunct to habits capitalizing on natural sun protection—such as seeking shade, spending less time outdoors during the hours when the sun is most direct, and wearing protective clothing. According to Dr. Guerry, sunscreens "are certainly likely to protect you from melanoma and nonmelanoma skin cancers, and they can play an integral part in keeping your skin healthy and young-appearing. But they don't substitute for sensible avoidance of excessive sun exposure. They should not be used simply to increase your sun-worshiping hours."

Sunscreens do help. A study conclusively showing their positive effects was done in Australia by Dr. Robin Marks. As reported in the *Skin Cancer Foundation Journal* in 1994, half the study participants wore plain cream without any sunscreen ingredients, and the other group applied lotion with a sun protection factor (SPF) of 17, effective against both UV-B and UV-A. Both groups were educated about avoiding excessive exposure to the intense Australian summer sun. The participants who applied the sunscreen had many fewer new solar keratoses, or small, flat, red, flaky growths on the skin that can be precursors to nonmelanoma skin cancers. Not only that, but those participants' existing keratoses seemed to disappear or stop growing.[12]

Sorting Out the Sun Protection Lotions   What is the best sunscreen lotion to wear? There are two basic types: some contain chemicals to absorb ultraviolet radiation, and others rely on particles of titanium dioxide or zinc oxide to block or scatter the light. The latter products are supposedly chemical-free but in fact contain inert chemicals. Some products are a combination of the two types. For some people, the disadvantage of titanium dioxide or zinc oxide is that until you wash the stuff off, your skin is an unattractive whitish color. Now micronized versions are available that break down the ingredients into tiny particles that blend in nicely with lighter skin colors.

You can take the SPF rating as an initial guide. The SPF measures the ability of a product to reduce the amount of UV-B radiation penetrating the skin. A sun protection factor of 10 reduces UV-B penetration by 90 percent, SPF 20 by 95 percent, and SPF 30 by 97 percent. Some feel that the SPF is not accurate: because a standardized measurement system for UV-A does not yet exist, the rating does not register the ability to block UV-A radiation.

You can't put a base of SPF 7 lotion on and then an SPF 15 sunscreen on top of it and expect them to add up to a protection factor of 22. Instead, the protection factor will be the higher of the two ratings (in this case 15). Most people don't use enough sunscreen to get effective protection. Food and Drug Administration guidelines suggest one ounce of cream for each application; you can assume that a bottle of sunscreen lotion will provide eight applications. You should apply your sunscreen at least forty-five minutes before going out into the sun, to allow for better bonding to the skin. Reapply sunscreen after going into the water: rarely will the protectant maintain its efficacy after you've been swimming.

Look for a product that specifies that it is a "broad spectrum" screen against both UV-B and UV-A. Better yet, choose a product that received a favorable rating in the May 1995 issue of *Consumer Reports* (or an update). The magazine tested sun protection lotions and rated them according to their water resistance and success in protecting against both UV-A and UV-B.[13]

Dr. Guerry generally recommends an SPF 15 but recognizes that SPFs of 30 and up are appropriate for the sun-sensitive. He reminds people to use the SPF number cautiously as a guideline to exposure time.

The UV Index   In July 1994, following much groundwork by the National Oceanic and Atmospheric Administration, the Environmental Protection Agency, and the Centers for Disease Control and Prevention, the UV index was inaugurated. A coalition of medical, environmental, and public health groups then vigorously promoted its use. In fifty-eight major cities now, the UV-B intensity can be predicted along with the weather. (If it isn't reported in your area, call the local weather service.) In Canada and England the index is updated daily on the basis of changes observed in the ozone layer.

The index predicts what the UV-B radiation will be in each participating city at "solar noon," when the sun is at its highest and its rays have the least distance to travel through

Figure 27. The UV Index

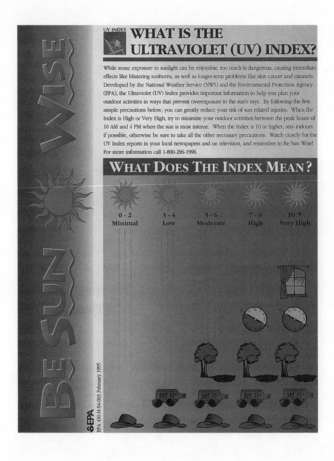

the atmosphere. To understand what the ratings mean and how to plan your activities according to the UV index, see Figure 27. Remember to take protective measures against the sun even when the index shows an acceptable level of radiation.

Sensible Sun Tips   In general, seeking shade, wearing protective clothing, generously applying a broad-spectrum sunscreen, and following the UV index forecast to avoid sunlight during peak hours can help you avoid damaging sun exposure. Remember that the shorter the shadow you cast, the greater your risk from sun exposure. Go to special lengths to protect your children from the sun; their skin is especially vulnerable to damage, and sunburns in childhood increase the risk of melanoma in adulthood.

- Before six months of age, children should have little direct exposure to the sun. Keep toddlers out of the sun during hours of peak intensity by planning outdoor activities outside these hours.
- Since children tend to imitate their parents (until they become teens), set a good example by covering them and yourself and avoiding outdoor activities during hours of prime intensity, ideally the three hours before and after solar noon.
- Don't patronize tanning salons.
- During times of intense sun, wear protective clothing, preferably in tight weaves. If you can see through the cloth when it is held up to light, then it probably offers inadequate protection. The sun protection factor for a typical t-shirt is only 6—and much lower when the shirt gets wet.
- Don't forget your head. Wear a wide-brimmed hat, with at least a four-inch brim all the way around. (*Don't wear a baseball cap backward!*) Make sure your sunscreen covers your ears and your neck up to the hairline.
- Protect your skin even on cloudy days. Clouds let most of the UV light pass through. Beach umbrellas and other shading devices offer only partial protection, because sand reflects a great deal of UV light.

- Apply a heavy, even coat of sunscreen lotion forty-five minutes before you go out, and reapply it frequently on humid days and when you'll be swimming or sweating a lot—even if the product is supposedly waterproof.
- Protect yourself with sunscreen when skiing too. Snow reflects more radiation, and the intensity of the sun's rays increases at high altitudes.
- Be cautious about using certain prescription drugs that increase sun sensitivity, such as some acne medications, antibiotics like doxycycline or tetracycline, and some diuretics. (Check with your pharmacist.)
- Don't consume alcohol and sit in the sun—you might fall asleep and get burned.
- "Bottled tans" are safe to use, but they don't provide any protection from the sun.
- Be aware that insect repellents, especially those containing DEET, dramatically reduce the effectiveness of your sunscreen lotion.

The aim of this chapter (and the book) is to inform you about melanoma and sun protection. But we shouldn't overreact to our environmental predicament. "As we manage our risks and those of our children," Dr. Guerry advises, "common sense should prevail. After all, we can't raise our children in the basement and overreact to the possibility of their or our getting skin cancer. So as with all the other things we do in life that are risky, *moderation* is the key."

Appendix A
Staging System for Melanoma

Malignant Melanoma of the Skin (Excluding Eyelid)

C44.0 Skin of lip, NOS	C51 Vulva
C44.2 External ear	
C44.3 Skin of other and unspecified parts of face	C60 Penis
C44.4 Skin of scalp and neck	C63.2 Scrotum
C44.5 Skin of trunk	
C44.6 Skin of upper limb and shoulder	
C44.7 Skin of lower limb and hip	
C44.8 Overlapping lesion of skin	
C44.9 Skin, NOS	

Malignant melanomas are most common in fair-skinned persons, often with a history of chronic sun exposure. They can occur in any skin area, including the palms, soles, and nail beds. Rarely, melanomas may arise in other sites, such as the mucous membranes of the oral cavity, nasopharynx, vagina, urethra, and anal canal. Melanomas may also arise from the pigmented tissues of the eye and from giant hairy nevi. In some cases of disseminated disease, a primary lesion may not be found. Melanomas can be transmitted from mother to infant during pregnancy. Early detection and treatment of incipient melanomas have resulted in a significant decrease in the mortality from this disease. The staging classification outlined in this chapter applies only to melanomas arising in the skin. These tumors are staged histologically by measuring the depth of penetration into the underlying dermis or subcutis and by a statement on the level of invasion, with the cutaneous anatomic structures used as reference.

ANATOMY

Primary Site.   The great majority of melanomas arise from the pigmented melanocytes located in the basal layer of the epidermis. The tumor often develops from a pre-existing pigmented lesion, although some arise from apparently normal skin. Melanomas are found on all skin surfaces. The tumor may grow into the dermis (nodular type) or spread horizontally along the skin (superficial spreading type). Multiple primary tumors may occur.

Regional Lymph Nodes.   The regional lymph nodes depend on the location of the primary tumor. Regional nodes are as follows:

Unilateral Tumors

Head and neck	Ipsilateral preauricular, submandibular, cervical, and supraclavicular lymph nodes
Thorax	Ipsilateral axillary lymph nodes
Arm	Ipsilateral epitrochlear and axillary lymph nodes
Abdomen, loins, and buttocks	Ipsilateral inguinal lymph nodes
Leg	Ipsilateral popliteal and inguinal lymph nodes
Anal margin and perianal skin	Ipsilateral inguinal lymph nodes

With tumors in the boundary zones between the above, the lymph nodes pertaining to the regions on both sides of the boundary zone are considered regional lymph nodes. The following 4 cm-wide bands are considered as boundary zones:

Between (Right/left)	*Along* (Midline)
Head and neck/thorax	Claviculo-acromion-upper shoulder blade edge

Thorax/arm	Shoulder-axilla-shoulder
Thorax/abdomen, loins, and buttocks	Front: Middle between navel and costal arch
	Back: Lower border of thoracic verte-brae (mid-transverse-axis)
Abdomen, loins, and buttock/leg	Groin-trochanter-gluteal sulcus

Iliac nodes are considered sites of distant metastasis and should be coded as M1.

Lesions arising in the midtransverse axis of the trunk at a level between the umbilicus and the lower costal margin anteriorly and extending laterally to the posterior level between the tenth thoracic spine (T10) and the first lumbar spine (L1) may spread with equal propensity to either contralateral or ipsilateral (or both) axillary or inguinal nodes.

Metastatic Sites.   Melanomas can metastasize widely. No organ or tissue is exempt. In some cases, metastatic deposits may not become apparent for years. Melanomas commonly involve skin, subcutaneous tissues, lymph nodes, liver, bone, lung, brain, and visceral organs.

For staging purposes, two sub-M categories, identified as "a" and "b," are included. Metastasis to the skin, subcutaneous tissue, or lymph nodes beyond the site of the primary lymph node drainage is considered M1a. Metastasis to other distant sites—often referred to as visceral metastasis—is considered M1b. This distinction is based on the more favorable response to therapy by patients with skin or subcutaneous metastases only.

DEFINITION OF TNM

Both the level of invasion and the maximum thickness determine the T classification and should be recorded. In case of discrepancy between tumor thickness and level, the pT category is based on the less favorable finding.

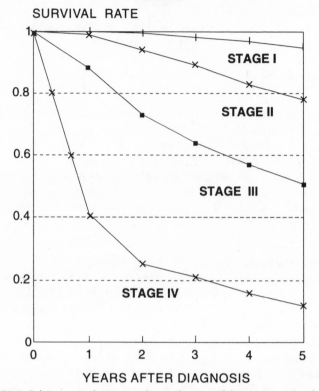

Survival According to AJCC Stage:
Melanoma

Fig. 24-1. Relative survival rates according to the stage of disease. Data taken from 8,479 patients who were diagnosed between 1977 and 1982. Patients are listed in the Surveillance, Epidemiology, and End Results Program of the National Cancer Institute. Stage I represents 4,286 patients; Stage II, 3,328; Stage III, 649; and Stage IV, 216.

Satellite lesions or subcutaneous nodules more than 2 cm from the primary tumor but not beyond the site of the primary lymph node drainage are considered in-transit metastases and are listed under the N categories.

The extent of tumor is classified after excision.

Primary Tumor (pT)

pTX   Primary tumor cannot be assessed

pTO   No evidence of primary tumor

pTis   Melanoma *in situ* (atypical melanocytic hyperplasia, severe melanocytic dysplasia), not an invasive lesion (Clark's Level I)

pT1   Tumor 0.75 mm or less in thickness and invading the papillary dermis (Clark's Level II)

pT2   Tumor more than 0.75 mm but not more than 1.5 mm in thickness and/or invades to the papillary-reticular dermal interface (Clark's Level III)

pT3   Tumor more than 1.5 mm but not more than 4 mm in thickness and/or invades the reticular dermis (Clark's Level IV)

     pT3a   Tumor more than 1.5 mm but not more than 3 mm in thickness

     pT3b   Tumor more than 3 mm but not more than 4 mm in thickness

pT4   Tumor more than 4 mm in thickness and/or invades the subcutaneous tissue (Clark's Level V) and/or satellite(s) within 2 cm of the primary tumor

     pT4a   Tumor more than 4 mm in thickness and/or invades the subcutaneous tissue

     pT4b   Satellite(s) within 2 cm of the primary tumor

Regional Lymph Nodes (N)

NX   Regional lymph nodes cannot be assessed

N0   No regional lymph node metastasis

N1   Metastasis 3 cm or less in greatest dimension in any regional lymph node(s)

N2   Metastasis more than 3 cm in greatest dimension in any regional lymph node(s) and/or in-transit metastasis

     N2a   Metastasis more than 3 cm in greatest dimension in any regional lymph nodes

     N2b   In-transit metastasis

     N2c   Both (N2a and N2b)

Distant Metastasis (M)

MX   Presence of distant metastasis cannot be assessed
M0   No distant metastasis
M1   Distant metastasis
     M1a   Metastasis in skin or subcutaneous tissue or lymph
               node(s) beyond the regional lymph nodes
     M1b   Visceral metastasis

Note: In-transit metastasis involves skin or subcutaneous tissue
more than 2 cm from the primary tumor not beyond the regional
lymph nodes.

STAGE GROUPING

Stage 0	pTis	N0	M0
	pT1	N0	M0
Stage I	pT1	N0	M0
	pT2	N0	M0
Stage II	pT3	N0	M0
	pT4	N0	M0
Stage III	Any pT	N1	M0
	Any pT	N2	M0
Stage IV	Any pT	Any N	M1

BIBLIOGRAPHY

1. Balch CM, Murad TM, Soong SJ, et al: A multifactorial analysis of
   melanoma: Prognostic histopathological features comparing
   Clark's and Breslow's staging lesions. Ann Surg 188:732–742, 1978

2. Breslow A: Thickness, cross-sectional areas and depth of invasion
   in the prognosis of cutaneous melanoma. Ann Surg 172:902–908,
   1970

3. Breslow A: Prognosis in cutaneous melanoma: Tumor thickness as
   a guide to treatment. Pathol Annu Part 1:1–20, 1980

4. Clark WH Jr: The histogenesis and biological behavior of primary
   malignant melanoma of the skin. Cancer Res 29:705–717, 1969

5. Kopf AW, Rodriquez-Sains RS, Rigel DS, et al: "Small" melanomas:
   Relation of prognostic variables to diameter of superficial spreading melanomas. J Dermatol Surg Oncol 8:765–770, 1982

Appendix B
Resources

─────────────────────────────

Computer Sources

American Academy of Dermatology

http://www.aad.org
Provides information on skin cancer.

American Cancer Society

http://www.cancer.org
Targets the most common cancers. Designed for patient education, this site offers the latest cancer statistics.

Anti-Cancer Council of Victoria (Australia)

www.auscharity.org

Cancer Care

http://www.cancercareinc.org
Provides a range of Web-based telephone services, including patient counseling, social services, local physician referrals, and financial assistance. The organization that produces it is supported by educational grants and private contributions.

CANCERLIT Topic Searches

http://cancernet.nci.nih.gov/canlit/canlit.htm
Appears monthly. The typical entry in this citation collection includes the title, author, source, and abstract of a recently published article.

Cansearch

http://www.access.digex.net/mkragen/index.html
Sponsored by the National Coalition for Cancer Survivorship, a not-for-profit support organization, this site brings together psychosocial resources for cancer patients and their families and also offers a guide to clinical trials.

Centers for Disease Control (CDC)

http://www.cdc.gov/publications.htm
Provides information on cancer prevention and control.

Environmental Protection Agency, Sunwise Program

http://www.epa.gov/ozone

Healthfinder

www.healthfinder.gov
Public health officials are calling this new Web site an easy entry point to trustworthy health information. The federal government had the site set up because consumers have difficulty weeding out faulty health information published on the Web.

Living with Cancer (Self-Help Group), Better Health and Medical Forum

Access through America Online. This forum meets on Sundays at 7:00 P.M. EST.

National Cancer Institute Cancer Centers Program

http://cancernet.nci.nih.gov/global/glo_pt.htm#nci-designated
This page lists the e-mail addresses, phone numbers, and Web sites of more than fifty sanctioned NCI Cancer Centers across the country. Substantial collections of reliable resources for patients and physicians can be found at these sites, such as those of the Johns Hopkins Oncology Center and the Memorial Sloan-Kettering Cancer Center.

Oncolink

http://www.oncolink.upenn.edu
This service provides late-breaking news and background information about cancer treatments, support groups, and educational information, twenty-four hours a day.

Physician's Data Query (PDQ)

http://cancernet.nci.hih.gov/pdq.htm
Updated monthly, PDQ is a service of the National Cancer Institute that provides answers to both patients' and doctors' questions regarding research, treatment, supportive care, screening, and investigational drugs. Also contains up-to-date information regarding prevention, early detection, and treatment that can be found on the Net. It is open to the general public but requires obtaining a member identification number and paying a fee.

Helpful Organizations

AUSTRALIA
Anti-Cancer Council of Victoria
1 Rathdone St.
Carlton South
Victoria 3053
tel.: 03-9279-1111

ENGLAND
Cancerlink
11–21 Northdown St
London N1 9BN
e-mail: cancerlink@canlink.demon.co.uk

FRANCE
Ecout Cancer
La Ligue National Contre le Cancer
1 avenue de la Grande Armée
75116 Paris

IRELAND
Irish Cancer Society
5 N Umberland Rd
Dublin No. 4

NETHERLANDS
Nederlandse Kankerbestrijving
Konigin Wilhemina Fonds
International Dutch Cancer Society
8 Sophialaan
1075 LBr Amsterdam

SCOTLAND
Cancerlink
9 Castle Terrace
Edinburgh EH1 2DP

Cancer Information Helpline (UK)
tel.: 0800 132905

UNITED STATES
Wellness Community
2716 Ocean Park Blvd.
Suite 1040
Santa Monica, CA 90405
tel.: 310-314-2555
fax: 310-314-2555

American Cancer Society
1599 Clifton Rd. NE
Atlanta, GA 30329
tel.: 800-ACS-2345

Publications

Helping Hand (melanoma support newsletter)
26 Belmont St.
Portland, ME 04101

Melanoma Letter
The Skin Cancer Foundation
245 Fifth Ave
Suite 2402
New York, NY 10016
For physicians (published quarterly), about the latest advances
in melanoma treatment.

The Skin Cancer Foundation publishes a multitude
of useful sources on melanoma. Write for further
information.

Melanoma Update
MSKCC, Box 421
1275 York Avenue
New York, NY 10021

Support Groups and Residential Programs
for Coping with Cancer

Commonweal
P.O. Box 316
Bolinas, CA 94924
tel.: 415-868-0970

Life After Cancer
121 Sherwood Rd.
Asheville, NC 28803
tel.: 704-252-4106
Support for those in or out of treatment

Nevus Network
2585 Treehouse Dr.
Lake Ridge, VA 22192
tel.: 703-492-0253
Support group for people with giant birth marks or garment nevi (see listings for the Wellness Community and American Cancer Society, which also provide support groups).

Outward Bound
tel. (gen. info.): 800-243-8520
(school): 800-643-4462

Simonton Cancer Center
P.O. Box 890
Pacific Palisades, CA 90272
tel.: 800-338-2360

Transportation

The following groups work to provide transportation for cancer patients who receive treatment at a distance from their homes:

Air Care Alliance, tel.: 800-296-1217
Corporate Angels Network, tel.: 914-328-1313

Suggested Reading

Charles Balch et al. *Cutaneous Melanoma,* 2nd ed. (Philadelphia: Lippincott Company, 1992). A comprehensive medical text on melanoma. Look for the latest edition.

Halvorson-Boyd, Hunter. *Dancing in Limbo* (San Francisco: Jossey-Bass, 1995). Written by a melanoma patient and a cancer patient;

addresses in a refreshing way the psychological issues that cancer patients face.

LeVert, Suzanne. *When Someone You Love Has Cancer* (New York: Dell Publishing, 1995). Hands-on book for the caregiver, including treatment of symptoms and hospice information.

Nessim, Susan, and Ellis, Judith. *Cancervive* (Boston: Houghton Mifflin, 1991). Also written by cancer survivors; addresses insurance as well as psychological issues.

Hotlines

The National Cancer Institute's Cancer Information Service hotline, tel.: 800-4-CANCER (funded by your tax dollars), usually operates out of your regional cancer center. Your doctor can reach the PDQ Search Service for Health Professionals at 800-345-3300. Outside the United States call 313-831-8292.
E-mail: pdqsearch@icicc.nci.nih.gov

EPA toll-free hotline, tel.: 800-296-1996

Melanoma Hotline, tel: 1-800-237-4724. Another service for doctors and patients. Nurses and social workers will answer questions regarding melanoma and treatment options. This hotline operates out of the University of Pittsburgh Cancer Institute Melanoma Center and is supported in part by the large pharmaceutical company Schering-Plough Corporation, makers of interferon alfa-2b.

Glossary

Actinic keratosis   Small, scaly red patch caused by sun exposure; potential precancer of the nonmelanoma type.

Adjuvant therapy   Treatment offered in addition to the surgical removal of melanoma (for instance). Generally, it affects the whole body and is designed to kill disease that may have traveled to other parts of the body even before the primary tumor or diseased lymph nodes were recognized and removed.

Basal cell carcinoma   One of two most common kinds of nonmelanoma cancer. It almost never metastasizes and is made up of the cells at the bottom layer of the epidermis that give rise to keratinocytes.

Biopsy   Surgical removal of a sample of tissue for examination under the microscope.

Carcinogen   Chemical, physical, or biological agent that causes cancer.

CAT or CT scan   X-ray procedure in which a computer produces detailed pictures of areas inside the body.

Congenital nevi   Moles that are present at birth, sometimes called birthmarks.

Dermis   The layer of skin directly beneath the epidermis.

Dermatopathologist   Physician who has special training in diagnosing disease on the basis of microscopic examination of the skin.

Dysplastic nevi Moles associated with an increased risk of melanoma. Larger than ordinary moles, they are flat or have a flat part, and have indistinct or fuzzy borders and often uneven coloration.

Epidermis The outermost layer of skin.

Excisional biopsy A biopsy to take all of a tumor that is in evidence.

Incisional biopsy A biopsy done with a knife that samples only a part of a lesion.

Interferon Type of protein produced by the immune system.

Interleukin-2 Type of protein molecule produced by lymphocytes that activates other lymphocytes in the immune system.

Lesion Well-defined, localized abnormality within an organ—e.g., a pigmented growth on the skin.

Lymphocyte Type of white blood cell that plays an important part in immune reactions.

Lymph gland, lymph node Small bean-shaped organs located in the lymphatic system.

Lymphoscintigraphy Technique of injecting a small amount of radioactive material near the site of a primary melanoma and then scanning different lymph node areas (armpits and groin for example) to see which group(s) of nodes "light up."

Melanocytes Cells located primarily at the bottom of the epidermis whose transfer of pigment to other cells is responsible in part for skin and hair color.

Metastasis Spread of cancer cells from one part of the body to another.

Nevus (plural *nevi*) Mole.

Pathology Science of diagnosing disease by such methods as microscopic analysis of tissue.

Pigmented lesion Skin spot that has color—brown, black, or blue.

Primary tumor or site Initial tumor or the body site where it forms.

Punch biopsy Biopsy in which a cookie cutter–like instrument is used to cut out a core of tissue.

Regional perfusion therapy Therapy in which a whole limb is infused with cancer-killing drugs. The drugs are introduced into the artery supplying the limb and are taken out through the vein. The technique may be used for melanoma when there are multiple skin metastases that are apparently confined to the arm or leg that was the site of the primary tumor.

Radial growth phase   Earliest step in the development of melanoma, in which the disease is confined to the epidermis or barely penetrates the dermis. No cluster of melanoma cells forms and no metastases result.

Seborrheic keratosis   Benign skin lesion associated with aging and sun exposure; not precancerous.

Shave biopsy   Biopsy done by shaving off a piece of skin with a sterile razor blade.

Squamous cell cancer   One of the two common kinds of non-melanoma skin cancer, a malignancy that seldom metastasizes and is made up of keratinocytes in the epidermis.

Subcutis, subcutaneous tissue   Layer of fat located under the dermis.

Stage (of cancer)   Measure of the extent of a malignancy, arrived at by examining features of the primary tumor and searching for evidence of metastasis.

Tumorigenic   Having the capacity to produce spherical collections of cancer cells.

UV-A and UV-B rays   Different wavelengths of ultraviolet light. Both are implicated in skin cancer, skin aging, and sunburn.

Vertical growth phase   Step in the development of melanoma in which the disease shows evidence of growth as a lump in the dermis (see *tumorigenic,* above). This phase of melanoma may metastasize.

Notes

Chapter 1 Close Encounters with Melanoma
1 Anthony Hecht, *The Transparent Man* (New York: Alfred Knopf, 1990).

Chapter 2 What Is Melanoma?
1 Charles Balch et al., *Cutaneous Melanoma*, 2nd ed. (Philadelphia: Lippincott, 1992), 6.

2 "Back in the U.S. There Was a Tide," in *American Decades: 1920–1929* (Detroit: Gale Research Press, 1994), 150.

3 Wallace Clark, "The Skin," in John Farber and Emanuel Rubin, eds., *Pathology* (Philadelphia: Lippincott, 1988).

4 Ibid.

5 Karen Shideler, "This Type of Melanoma Killed Bob Marley," and "When Ultraviolet Rays of Sunshine Become Ultraviolent: Skin Cancers," *Philadelphia Inquirer*, Aug. 1, 1994.

6 DuPont Guerry et al., "Lessons from Tumor Progression: The Invasive Radial Growth Phase of Melanoma Is Common, Incapable of Metastasis and Indolent," *Journal of Investigative Dermatology* 100 (1992): 3425–3455.

Chapter 3 Who Gets Melanoma and Why
1 W. Norris, "Eight Cases of Melanosis with Pathological and Therapeutical Remarks on That Disease" (London: Longman, Brown, Green, Longman and Roberts, 1857).

2 "Estimating Individual Risk for Developing Cutaneous Malignant Melanoma," a lecture presented in Oct. 1996, by Marianne

Berwick, assistant attending epidemiologist at Memorial Sloan-Kettering Cancer Center.

3   Patricia Ceballos et al., "Melanoma in Children," *New England Journal of Medicine* 12 (1995): 656–660.

4   Richard Gallagher et al., "The Epidemiology of Acquired Melanocytic Nevi," *Dermatoepidemiology* 13 (1995): 3.

5   Alfred Kopf et al., "Prospective Follow-Up for Malignant Melanoma in Patients with Atypical Moles (Dysplastic Nevus Syndrome)," *Journal of Dermatologic Surgery and Oncology* 17 (1991): 44–48.

6   Allan Halpern, "Melanoma Surveillance: The High-Risk Patient," *Skin Cancer Foundation Journal* (1992): 42.

7   Elizabeth Holly, Rosemary Cress, and David Ahn, "Cutaneous Melanoma in Women: Reproductive Factors and Oral Contraceptive Use," *American Journal of Epidemiology* 141 (1995): 943–950.

8   Rona McKie et al., "Lack of Effect of Pregnancy on Outcome of Melanoma," *Lancet* 337 (1991): 653–655.

9   Elizabeth Holly, Rosemary Cress, and David Ahn, "Cutaneous Melanoma in Women: Ovulatory Life, Menopause, and Use of Exogenous Estrogens," *Cancer Epidemiology, Biomarkers and Prevention* 3 (1994): 661–668.

10   Ibid.

11   C. Garbe, "Pregnancy, Hormone Preparations and Malignant Melanoma," *Hautarzt* [Dermatologist] 44 (1996): 347–352.

Chapter 4   Finding Early Melanoma

1   Guerry et al., "Lessons from Tumor Progression."

2   Marianne Berwick et al., "Screening for Cutaneous Melanoma by Skin Self-Examination," *Journal of the National Cancer Institute* 88 (1996): 17–23.

3   Rosemary Cress et al., "Cutaneous Melanoma in Women: Anatomic Distribution in Relation to Sun Exposure and Phenotype," *Cancer Epidemiology, Biomarkers and Prevention* 4 (1995): 831–836.

4   Barrie Casselieth et al., "Catalyst Symptoms in Malignant Melanoma," *Journal of General Internal Medicine* 2 (1987): 1–4.

5   Howard Koh et al. "Who Discovers Melanoma," *Journal of the American Academy of Dermatology* 26 (1992): 914–919.

6   Ibid.

7   Peggy Eastman, "CDC-Dermatologists Partnership Will Target Skin Cancer," *Oncology Times* (May 1996): 57.

8   Howard Koh, "Early Detection of Melanoma: An Ounce of Prevention May Be a Ton of Work," *Journal of the American Academy of Dermatology* (Apr. 1993): 644–646.

9   Howard Koh, general lecture on melanoma given at the hospital at the University of Pennsylvania, Oct. 1996.

Chapter 5   If You Have Melanoma

1   American Cancer Society, *Facts on Skin Cancer* (American Cancer Society, 1995).

2   Wallace Clark et al., "Model Predicting Survival in Stage I Melanoma Based on Tumor Progression," *Journal of the National Cancer Institute* 81 (1989): 369–375.

3   Lynn Schuchter et al., "A Prognostic Model for Predicting 10-Year Survival in Patients with Primary Melanoma," *Annals of Internal Medicine* 125 (Sept. 1996): 1893–1904.

4   Charles M. Balch et al., "Efficacy of an Elective Lymph Node Dissection of 1 to 4mm.-Thick Melanomas in Patients 60 Years of Age and Younger," *Annals of Surgery* 224 (1996): 255–266.

5   Donald Morton et al., "Management of Early Stage Melanoma by Intraoperative Lymphatic Mapping," *Surgical Oncology Clinics of America,* 1 (1992), 534.

Chapter 6   When Melanoma Metastasizes

1   John Kirkwood et al., "Interferon Alfa-2b Adjuvant Therapy of High-Risk Resected Cutaneous Melanoma: The Eastern Cooperative Oncology Group Trial," *Journal of Clinical Oncology* 14 (1996): 7–17.

2   Ian H. Krakoff, "Systemic Treatment of Cancer," *Cancer: A Cancer Journal for Clinicians* 46 (1996): 134–141.

3   Stephen Rosenberg, "Current Status of Vaccine Treatment of Melanoma," lecture given at the University of Pennsylvania Cancer Center, Nov. 8, 1996.

Chapter 7   Tending to Your Spirits

1   David Spiegel, "Effect of Psychosocial Treatment on Survival of Patients with Metastatic Breast Cancer," *Lancet* (Oct. 14, 1989): 888–890.

2   Fawzy Fawzy, "Malignant Melanoma: Effects of an Early Structured Psychiatric Intervention, Coping, and Affective State on

Recurrence and Survival, Six Years Later," *Archives of General Psychiatry* (Aug. 1990): 681–689.

Chapter 8 Prevention of Melanoma

1 "What's Melanoma?" survey reported in the *Washington Post,* June 13, 1996.

2 Anti-Cancer Council of Victoria, Australia, *SunSmart Program Outline, 1993–1996* (Anti-Cancer Council of Victoria: Victoria, n.d.).

3 Ibid.

4 Lois Losescher et al., "Public Education Projects in Skin Cancer," *Cancer* 75 (1995): 651–656.

5 Howard Koh, general lecture on melanoma given at the hospital at the University of Pennsylvania, Oct. 1996.

6 "What's Melanoma?" survey.

7 A quiz designed to bring home to teenagers the dangers of sun exposure appeared in the June 1996 issue of *Sassy Magazine,* pp. 68–70.

8 Anti-Cancer Council of Victoria, Australia, *SunSmart Program Outline.*

9 Eastman, "CDC-Dermatologists Partnership."

10 Howard Koh, general lecture on melanoma given at the hospital at the University of Pennsylvania, Oct. 1996.

11 Mark Jaffe, "Findings Mixed in Latest Report on Loss of Ozone," *Philadelphia Inquirer,* Oct. 12, 1994.

12 Robin Marks, "Daily Sunscreen Use Can Reduce the Risk of Skin Cancer," *Skin Cancer Foundation Journal* 12 (1994): 10.

13 "Putting Sunscreens to the Test," *Consumer Reports* (May 1995): 333–343.

Index

Page references in italics refer to illustrations.

Nev